L
D

THE L.A. DIET

JAMES J. KENNEY, Ph.D., R.D.
and
DIANE GRABOWSKI, M.N.S., R.D.

CB
CONTEMPORARY
BOOKS
CHICAGO · NEW YORK

Library of Congress Cataloging-in-Publication Data

Kenney, James J.
    The L.A. diet : the eating plan that raises your metabolism to
lose fat forever / James J. Kenney, Diane Grabowski.
        p.   cm.
    Includes index.
    1. Reducing diets.   2. High-carbohydrate diet.   3. Low-fat diet.
4. Food habits.   I. Grabowski, Diane.   II. Title.
ISBN 0-8092-4710-0
RM222.2.K448   1988
613.2'5—dc 19   88-250
                                                                CIP

Published by Contemporary Books, Inc.
180 North Michigan Avenue, Chicago, Illinois 60601
Manufactured in the United States of America
Library of Congress Catalog Card Number: 88-280
International Standard Book Number: 0-8092-4710-0

Published simultaneously in Canada by Beaverbooks, Ltd.
195 Allstate Parkway, Valleywood Business Park
Markham, Ontario L3R 4T8 Canada

CONTENTS

FOREWORD

James Kenney and Diane Grabowski have taken on a difficult task and come up with a serious, interesting, and eminently worthwhile approach to weight control. The ideas conveyed in this book are noteworthy and useful, not only for weight control but as a general guide to healthful eating. Dr. Kenney brings to this book many years of experience, both as a researcher and as a practitioner of the science and art of nutrition and dietetics. Unlike so many books on the subject of dieting and weight control, *The L.A. Diet* undergirds all its recommendations with the scientific data and their explanation.

Obesity, weight reduction, and weight control are among the most difficult and elusive areas that the nutritional and medical scientist has had to deal with in recent years. The failure rate among individuals who have followed countless other approaches is frighteningly high. The approach of reducing one's total fat intake and eating many small meals during the day has not been presented before in the clear, precise, and hands-on way in which it is outlined in *The L.A. Diet*. It is an interesting book, not only for those of us who desperately need practical help to solve a major physical and health problem, but also for the serious student in the nutritional and medical sciences.

Hans Fisher, Ph.D.
Department of Nutrition
Rutgers, The State University of
New Jersey

FOREWORD

Dr. Kenney's extensive new book provides a comprehensive analysis to the growing health concern of obesity. It reviews in detail the many health benefits of adopting a low-fat, high-complex-carbohydrate diet not the least of which is the safest and most effective weight control program devised since Nathan Pritikin first exposed the fallacies of the highly processed, high-fat American diet in his bestselling book *Live Longer Now* over ten years ago.

Dr. Kenney analyzes the growing body of scientific and clinical reports that deal with the impact of diet and other lifestyle factors on the accumulation of excess body fat. The comprehensive theory he puts forth in this book provides many insights into why other weight control programs are doomed to long-term failure and how the "grazing" lifestyle he describes offers a realistic solution to what has become one of this nation's most frustrating health problems.

We believe that *The L.A. Diet* offers a straightforward solution to obesity. It is for people who have tired of all the fad diets and nutritional gimmickry that offer more fantasy than fact and produce at best short-term success and long-term guilt. After you digest the hard facts in this book, you will be in control of your weight and your health.

Robert Pritikin
Director
Pritikin Research Foundation
Santa Barbara, California

Monroe Rosenthal, M.D.
Medical Director
Ocean View Medical Group
Santa Monica, California

THE
L.A.
DIET

INTRODUCTION: GRAZING VERSUS GORGING

Grazing has become a buzzword for a new style of dining that is revolutionizing America's eating habits. Three square meals a day are giving way to smaller but more frequent meals. Behind this grazing philosophy is a desire to fuse what in the past were two mutually exclusive attitudes about food. One focused only on the gustatory pleasure of eating without regard to the health consequences of those choices. The second focused primarily on food's impact on health, often with an emphasis on weight control.

This book explains how a grazing lifestyle can give you the best of both worlds. With the L.A. Diet Program you can have enjoyable meals and better health. You can lose weight and keep it off without feeling hungry and tired all the time. You will be able to eat more food more frequently—eating as much as you want—and still lose weight. Once you understand why you get fat, you will be able to control your weight. And you won't need any gimmicks or gadgets. You won't have to purchase any "magical" pills, powders, or potions.

This book provides everything you need to adopt L.A.'s grazing lifestyle for eating plenty of delicious food that will satisfy your appetite and help you reach—and stay at—the weight you desire.

Part I explains the principles behind the L.A. Diet Program: why you

1

get fat; why other diets haven't worked—and won't work—for you; why a low-calorie, low-fat, high-carbohydrate diet is the *only* way to work *with* your metabolism instead of against it to take weight off permanently; how exercise and occasional "cheating" will fit into your new lifestyle; and more.

Part II sets you on an unwavering course to better health and lifelong weight loss. It explains in practical terms how to fit six small meals into daily life versus the usual two or three large meals; how to stock your kitchen with useful equipment and nutritious, acceptable foods; how to balance those six meals for optimum intake of nutrients; what types of dishes to plan for breakfast, lunch, dinner, and snacks; and how to eat away from home without detouring from the L.A. Diet.

Part III is the recipe section of the book. Here you'll find a wealth of appetizers, light soups, salads, entrees, desserts, beverages, "munchies," and more. And to help you become a gourmet grazer, there's a chapter full of tips for making *nutritious* equal *delicious* plus recipes any party giver would be proud to offer to discriminating friends.

WHAT IS GRAZING?

According to Webster, *grazing* is defined as feeding on growing herbage. *Herbage,* in turn, is variously defined as grasses and the succulent parts of plants (that's vegetables). Animals that eat only vegetable matter are called *herbivores,* in contrast to *carnivores,* which feed primarily on the flesh of other animals. Human beings are primates, a family of mammals whose feeding style is often described as *foraging.* Foraging can be viewed as a specialized form of grazing to which all primates are physiologically adapted.

It is true that some monkeys and apes eat the flesh of other animals, but in their natural setting they consume primarily vegetable matter. Like our primate "cousins," we are grazers by nature. We pay a heavy price in terms of our health for going against our biological heritage. Mounting scientific and clinical evidence strongly indicates that human beings, in contrast to large carnivores, are not designed to gorge.

It's Not Nice to Try to Fool Mother Nature

What we are biologically was determined at our conception, and there is little we can do to change our genetic heritage. You can take man out of nature, but you cannot take the nature out of man. The L.A. Diet is based on the scientific appraisal of the nutritional needs of man.

If you have gotten most of your information about nutrition from best-selling books, magazine articles, health food store employees, and/or TV talk shows, you have been largely misinformed about how what you eat affects your health. What you get from these sources is a confusing blend of facts and fantasies. Unfortunately, usually the fantasies are much more appealing than the facts. If you are tired of going from one unrealistic weight-loss fantasy to another, you've found the right book. Unlike so many of its predecessors, the L.A. Diet is based on solid scientific research. This research forms the backbone of the grazing approach to permanent weight control.

THE KEYS TO SUCCESSFUL WEIGHT CONTROL

In order to control your weight and/or reduce your chances of developing a wide variety of diet-related health problems, you must have two things: motivation and accurate information. Either of these alone will not suffice. Misinformation about how diet affects body weight is so widespread that it is a wonder anyone ever succeeds in keeping off excess weight.

The few people who successfully control their weight by counting calories are doomed to chronic hunger, irritability, and fatigue. A few may succeed temporarily by doing Herculean amounts of exercise, but how many can keep this up for a lifetime? Most "succeed" by becoming so obsessive-compulsive about food that they have trouble dealing with the rest of life.

Self-starvation, binging and purging, and even "overeating" have been blamed on what psychologists term *eating disorders*. Psychologists and psychiatrists are increasingly diagnosing such eating disorders as anorexia and bulimia, which they treat with a variety of behavioral modification techniques. If the condition becomes life-threatening, they put you in a hospital and stick a tube in your arm.

People who become overweight because they fail to starve themselves or purge themselves after gorging on calorically dense foods are treated with "aversive therapy," surgery, and a variety of drugs. Now if you stop and think about all of these eating disorder "treatments," they begin to seem a lot more like punishments than treatments.

When You Are Out of Control, You Put Others in Charge

Most weight loss "therapies" work on the assumption that you are either too ignorant, too weak-willed, or too lazy to control your own body. Eventually most dieters come to accept these assumptions about themselves. Once you have accepted the idea that you cannot control your own body weight, you seek out others who share these assumptions about you. Enter the doctors, psychologists, and quacks. And in the name of "therapy," these people subject you to medication, surgery, aversive conditioning, or hypnosis. They staple your ears or stick pins in you (accupuncture). Is that torture of therapy? They staple your stomach or stick a balloon in it. Torture or therapy? They give you electric shocks and wire your mouth shut. They hypnotize you and criticize you until you do what they tell you. Brainwashing or therapy? They cut out your stomach and intestines. Therapy or mutilation? They starve you (fasting) or put you on nutritionally inadequate diets and make you go to bed without dessert. Therapy or punishment? Are the drugs they use therapy or poisons? Do they make you healthier or more unhealthy? Is the "cure" worse than the disease?

The quacks sell you gimmicks and gadgets, pills, powders, and "magical" potions—and they all seem to work for everyone but you. Unfortunately, if you are like most overweight people, you're more likely to blame yourself than a useless product.

This book will explain why there are no simple solutions to weight control. If you've tried any of these "guaranteed" methods, you probably weren't satisfied with the results for long. After all of these failures, you probably have asked, "What is wrong with me?" when you should have asked, "What is wrong with *them?*" There is absolutely no scientific evidence to back the claims made for any of these gadgets and pills. There are no "secrets" to losing weight permanently. It takes knowing what to do and how to do it. And it takes a desire to change.

INFORMATION + MOTIVATION = CONTROL

Controlling your body weight (or anything else) requires accurate information as well as the motivation or desire to use that information to make the necessary changes. In order to control anything you must first understand how it works. Nevertheless, the vast majority of people who try to lose weight do not first take the time to learn how their body fat level is regulated. You need to know how your activity level and what you eat interacts with inherited characteristics to determine how much body fat you will store. Since there is no way to change your chromosomes, you must change your activity level and/or your diet in order to control your weight. The scientific evidence has proven beyond a reasonable doubt that the L.A. Diet described in this book is the only way to control your weight permanently by shedding excess body fat.

Why Willpower Won't Work

The big mistake made by most psychologists and dietitians involved in weight counseling has been the working assumption that all you have to do to lose weight is to count calories and eat less. On a very superficial level this is correct; we know that cutting calories causes weight loss.

We also know that simply cutting calories causes your metabolic rate to slow down, because your "metabolic furnace" is receiving less fuel. You end up cold, hungry, and lethargic because your body needs far more fuel (calories) to run efficiently than it is getting.

In the short run, the intellect can go against the body's real needs. But, in reality, the unconscious drive states such as hunger, thirst, and the need to stay warm determine what you are. In a sense, *you are what you need.* In the long run it is, therefore, self-destructive to deny your biological needs. Self-denial leads to self-destruction. An extreme example of how self-denial leads to self-destruction is anorexia nervosa. It illustrates in a tragic way how destructive it can be to continually go against your biological drive states.

"Dieting" by counting calories and consciously restricting your food intake is self-destructive because it is need denial. It is a no-win situation. The appetite control mechanism in your brain is constantly driving you to eat more than your intellect knows you can and still stay thin. There can never be a resolution to this conflict. When you simply cut calories without changing the composition of your diet, you create a conflict between the conscious self and the unconscious drive state. This conflict leads to chronic frustration because there is no resolution. Frustration and confusion undermine your intellect (or willpower) and ultimately cause you to overeat or binge. Between binges you live in constant fear of going "out of control." But you really are not going out of control. What is happening is that control is shifting between your conscious self and your unconscious drive state, which are constantly at odds.

Self-Denial Leads to Self-Hatred

You begin to hate yourself for not being able to keep the weight off. You should be thankful your unconscious drive state is winning the battle. Self-denial or need denial leads to self-destruction. If you hate yourself enough, anorexia nervosa can result.

Success Is Failure

Do not lament your lack of willpower; it has the power to destroy you only when it conflicts with your real needs. Do not curse yourself for being a failure. Your will to live is simply stronger than your desire to conform. Trying to be what you are not leads to self-destruction. Succeeding at being what you are not weakens your will to live because it conflicts with your desire to meet your biological needs. You need enough fuel to keep warm and maintain normal metabolic function. Without it you will be cold, hungry, and run-down. It is the self-hatred associated with the failed irrational attempts to lose weight and keep it off that leads many dieters to the quacks, psychologists, pill pushers, and surgeons.

If you read this book thoroughly, you will realize you are fat because you *eat* fat, not because you are weak-willed, stupid, or lazy. Once you understand how fat makes you fat and why whatever warms you up slims you down, you are on your way to rationally controlling your weight; you can begin to alter your diet and activity level to control your level of body fat. This, of course, means changing ingrained eating habits. However, once you have adopted the L.A. Diet, you will feel better about yourself, not detached and alienated from your biological being. There will be no unresolvable conflict between your unconscious drive state and your intellect. The L.A. Diet puts them in harmony.

This is not to say that changing to the L.A. Diet will be easy. You will be tempted by some of your old favorite fatty foods from time to time, especially when conflict and stress in other parts of your life make you feel like retreating or regressing to your old habits. But with the L.A. Diet there is a light at the end of the tunnel. The longer you go without gorging, the easier it gets. Calorie-counting gorgers are constantly being driven to eat more. Grazers will be *tempted* to cheat, but they will not be *driven* to cheat on this weight control plan. With grazing you eat as much as you want. You don't count calories, and your metabolic rate does not drop. You do not chill easily and will have plenty of energy.

Once you appreciate the difference between being tempted and being driven, you can begin to understand why the L.A. Diet offers a permanent solution to the problem of weight control. Whereas other diet plans set up an unresolvable conflict between your intellect and your biological drive state, grazing puts you in control. You may be tempted, but you will never be driven to fail. Rather than looking for someone or something to control what you believed was an irrational desire to "overeat," you will be grazing to your heart's content.

GORGING IS NATURAL—IF YOU'RE A BEAR

It is not natural to spend most of your waking hours focusing on food. In nature, apes and monkeys do not get fat, and they do not count calories.

Gorging, in contrast to grazing, best describes the current eating habits of most Americans and Europeans. In the natural world, lions, tigers, wolves, grizzly bears, and polar bears are the quintessential gorgers. It is natural for these large predators to gorge. In this book, *gorging* refers to consuming unnatural foods or consuming natural foods in unnatural amounts.

Unnatural foods are those that have been altered by processing. Potatoes are natural, but potato chips are unnatural no matter what the label says. Refined fats and oils and refined sugar are not natural. The highly concentrated calories in these foods make them gorging foods despite their origin. It makes little difference nutritionally whether the calories in plants are concentrated in an animal's body or by the food processor's machinery. The result is a concentrated source of calories.

There is nothing unnatural about a little fish, meat, or poultry. But it *is* unnatural for these foods to make up a large part of our diet. Large predatory animals, like the grizzly bear and lion, are *metabolically geared* for a gorging lifestyle. Their very survival often depends on fattening up during times of plenty so that they can survive the long cold winters of Alaska or the hot dry summers of the Serengeti Plain when food is scarce. *It is their nature, not ours.*

In the wild, gorillas, chimpanzees, and other primates are very lean. They do not get clogged arteries, diabetes, or high blood pressure. But when primates are fed a typical Western diet, most succumb to all of the above and become obese. The scientific evidence clearly indicates that physiologically and biochemically human beings are designed more for grazing than gorging. It is our shift from grazing to gorging that is causing most of the serious diseases that afflict Western man, including obesity.

THE PRINCIPLES BEHIND THE L.A. DIET

The good news is that scientific research in the field of nutrition has made it possible to develop a rational approach to weight control and total health. Unlike many of its predecessors, this is not just another fad diet book designed to cash in on the hopes and fantasies of the millions of desperate, overweight Americans. It explains why fad diets, behavioral techniques, calorie counting, and diet pills do not offer a long-term solution to the problem of weight control and why excess body fat is the natural result of adopting a typical (but unnatural) Western lifestyle.

Part I of this book synthesizes the latest theories as to why many people gain excessive amounts of body fat into one revolutionary new concept. That concept, the foundation of the L.A. Diet Program, explains what causes obesity and why grazing is the key element in getting rid of excess body fat permanently.

A key to this conceptual breakthrough deals with the interaction of body temperature regulation with body fat regulation. We know that a specialized organ within the brain (the hypothalamus) regulates both body temperature and appetite, and it seems that anything that consistently warms the body reduces the body's need for fat. Body fat serves both as a source of fuel to keep you warm and as insulation that helps to keep you warm when your metabolic furnace isn't producing enough heat due to a shortage of other sources of fuel.

Whatever Warms You Up Slims You Down

In simple terms, you will learn why *whatever warms you up slims you down*. In order to get rid of excess body fat and keep it off, you must do those things that tend to increase body temperature and reduce the need for stored fat. *More heat means less need for insulating body fat under your skin.* As we shall see, the L.A. Diet Program is the only safe and effective way to generate extra heat and reduce body fat without ending up tired, hungry, and/or cold most of the time. Chapter 2 explains how body temperature regulation influences body fat stores.

A High-Carbohydrate, Low-Fat Diet

Research has proven that the body produces much more heat when it metabolizes carbohydrates than when it metabolizes fats. Therefore, it makes sense that by grazing you will lower the amount of insulating body fat your body needs to stay warm. Why eating fat makes us fat is explained further in Chapter 3.

Less than 10 percent of the Japanese men 45–65 years of age are overweight, while 63 percent of American males the same age are overweight. The traditional Japanese diet is low in fat and high in carbohydrates, while the standard American diet is high in fat and much lower in carbohydrates. The L.A. Diet emphasizes low-fat foods such as fruits, vegetables, potatoes, and whole grain products.

Table 1 shows the differences in nutrient content between the L.A. Diet and the standard American diet. You can see that the L.A. Diet is

TABLE 1. A COMPARISON OF THE NUTRITIONAL COMPOSITION OF
THE L.A. DIET AND THE STANDARD AMERICAN DIET

Food Component	L.A. Diet	Standard American Diet
Fat (% of Calories)	5–10	35–45
Refined Carbohydrate (% of Calories)	<5	>35
Unrefined Carbohydrate (% of Calories)	>70	<15
Protein (% of Calories)	10–15	10–15
Alcohol (% of Calories)	0–3	5–10
Dietary Fiber (Grams/day)	>50	<15
Salt (Grams/day)	<4	>8

< indicates "less than"; > indicates "more than"

much lower in fat and much higher in carbohydrates. It is also much higher in unrefined carbohydrates and fiber.

Frequent Small Meals

Eating only one or two large high-fat meals a day can actually encourage your body to burn carbohydrates while storing that fat you want to get rid of. In contrast, eating smaller meals more frequently stokes the metabolic furnace, producing more heat. Again, being warm lowers your body's need for insulating body fat. In Chapter 2, you'll learn the role of body temperature regulation in weight control—why whatever warms you up slims you down.

Grazing Lowers Your "Set Point" for Body Fat

As we shall see, diets that do not consider the physiological basis for the accumulation of excess body fat are self-defeating. Unless you follow an eating plan that permanently reduces the amount of body fat needed to maintain body temperature and normal metabolic function, you will have an extra layer of body fat under your skin for insulation. This means that your level of body fat ("set point") will be maintained too high for optimal health. When you are below this set point for body fat, your metabolic rate is slowed and you feel tired, hungry, and cold.

Most people have trouble with being hungry, tired, and/or cold much of the time. This is why they are driven to "overeat" and regain any weight lost by fasting or counting calories. Simply cutting back on calories disrupts your body's fuel supply, which slows your metabolic rate. A slower metabolic rate means less heat is produced, so you chill more easily. A lack of metabolic fuel makes you feel hungry and lethargic.

The L.A. Diet Program is designed to permanently lower your body's physiological need for extra body fat. It will lower your set point for body fat. Understanding how dietary factors interact with an inherited predisposition to store excess body fat has enabled me to devise a plan for permanently shedding excess body fat. Since you cannot change your genes, adopting the L.A. Diet Program is the only way to permanently lower your body's need for extra (insulating) fat. The role of genetic factors in producing obesity is the subject of Chapter 1.

This program is designed to "turn down" your body's set point for body fat (thereby decreasing the need for insulation). By doing this, the L.A. Diet Program does not create a conflict between your conscious desire to weigh less and your brain's thermoregulatory mechanism. Since the regulation of body temperature also involves regulating hunger and satiety centers in the hypothalamus, adopting the L.A. Diet Program has two important effects: (1) it suppresses your appetite so that you won't want to eat as much, and (2) it maintains a normal metabolic rate on fewer calories so that you do not chill easily and feel hungry and run-down most of the time.

It is precisely because other dietary plans do not impact on your set point for body fat that these plans doom you to long-term failure before you start. They depend on your conscious willpower to control how much you eat. The more body fat you lose, the hungrier you get. The result is an unresolvable conflict between your intellect and your natural physiological makeup.

GRAZING FOR OPTIMAL HEALTH AND WEIGHT CONTROL

The lifestyle changes recommended in this book are just as important to your family and friends, regardless of their weight, as they are to you. The L.A. Diet is not a special diet for the obese but rather a healthy diet and lifestyle for virtually everyone. How this plan can contribute to overall health and longevity is the subject of Chapter 7. If your goal is to look, feel, and be healthy, the L.A. Diet is the only realistic solution to long-term weight control.

I
FACTS ABOUT PERMANENT WEIGHT LOSS

by James J. Kenney, Ph.D., R.D.

1
HEREDITY IS NOT DESTINY

There is mounting scientific evidence that the tendency to become obese is inherited. Indeed, the tendency to become obese apears to be more strongly dependent on genetic factors than heart disease, breast cancer, high blood pressure, or schizophrenia. Precisely how the tendency to become obese is inherited is not known, but research has proven beyond a reasonable doubt that most, if not all, overfat Americans had the misfortune of inheriting a set of chromosomes (which contain the genes or genetic material) from their parents that makes them more efficient at storing body fat than their leaner friends and relatives.

On the other hand, there are some people who burn fat so efficiently and store it so poorly that they stay lean even while gorging. Unfortunately, lean gorgers consuming a typical American diet rarely have contented hearts, because in most of them the blood vessels that feed the heart are becoming clogged with fatty cholesterol deposits. Indeed, one out of every five men will have a heart attack before his fiftieth birthday, and most of these men will be within 10 or 20 pounds of their "ideal" body weight. See Chapter 7 for more on this subject.

RESEARCH LINKING GENES
TO OBESITY IN HUMANS

Classical research linking genetic factors to excessive adiposity in people found that the incidence of obesity was only 14 percent in the offspring of lean parents. If one parent was obese, then about 40 percent of the children eventually become obese. When both parents were obese, 8 out of every 10 children became obese as adults. Other studies demonstrated that abdominal skin folds (a measure of subcutaneous fat) of children correlated closely with that of their parents.

Even when environmental factors (dietary lifestyle) were taken into account, much research has suggested that the amount and distribution of body fat a person has depends more on inherited characteristics than environmental factors. Studies involving adopted children and separated twins have shown that the children's body fat level correlated much more closely with that of their biological parents than that of their adoptive or foster parents. In these studies genetic influences, not diet, determined who got fat.

Table 1.1 shows the heritability estimates for obesity and several other medical conditions. (Heritability is simply a measure of how strongly a certain characteristic or trait is due to genes.)

TABLE 1.1. HERITABILITY OF OBESITY AND OTHER MEDICAL CONDITIONS

Condition	Hereditability Factor
Obesity at Age 20	.80
Obesity at Age 45	.64
Schizophrenia	.68
High Blood Pressure	.57
Alcoholism	.57
Cirrhosis of the Liver	.53
Epilepsy	.50
Coronary Artery Disease	.49
Breast Cancer	.45

JAMA, July 4, 1986 (Vol. 256, No. 1)

These lines of research prove beyond a reasonable doubt that, at the very least, the *tendency* to become obese is determined by inherited factors. It has also led to a lot of speculation that obesity is inevitable and inescapable for those unfortunate individuals who inherit "fat" genes.

However, as we will see in this chapter, heredity is *not* destiny. Many people inherit a tendency to develop high blood pressure, but they experience hypertension only when their diet is high in salt. Similarly, while many individuals inherit a tendency to become obese, only those who adopt a high-fat diet and are inactive actually become overfat.

Conversely, those who inherit "lean" genes may find that they never get fat, regardless of what and how much they eat. Such "lean" genes are not, however, a green light for gorging. The benefits derived from grazing are far more difficult to observe in a thin person than an obese person. Nevertheless, from the perspective of attaining optimal health, grazing is every bit as important to the genetically lean individual as the overfat person.

As you will see, what is inherited is a tendency to become overfat *only* when food is plentiful, accessible, high in fat, and low in fiber. This is, of course, the case for the great majority of people in the United States and most of Europe. Since almost everyone in these cultures is gorging, it is genetic factors that determine how much body fat an individual will store. In other words, given an environment that promotes obesity, only those who inherit a strong genetic resistance to storing extra body fat will remain fairly lean.

Nearly all of us inherit certain metabolic tendencies that may have survival value under some circumstances but can undermine our health and well-being under different conditions. The inherited tendency to become obese is a perfect example of this type of mixed blessing. The health hazards of excess body fat are many. Current estimates predict you lose at least one year of life for every 10 pounds of excess body fat.

FAT INCREASES SURVIVAL

Not that long ago, however, being obese actually increased one's chances of surviving the frequent famines that plagued most human cultures until recent years. People who stored a lot of fat during times of plenty had a better chance of surviving a year when the crops failed.

It is hard to imagine that "survival of the fittest" could ever be equated with "survival of the fattest." However, an average-weight person can survive about two months without food while a moderately obese individual can often survive for more than six months. So while you may curse your "fat" genes for making you fat, it is quite possible that your great-great-grandparents survived a famine or two precisely because they carried those genes. A lot of naturally thin people were never born because their forebears did not survive the potato famine in Ireland or some other prolonged food shortage in another region. It would appear that the laws of natural selection were selecting "fat genes" for countless generations in many cultures. The legacy of this natural selection is a large percentage of "fat genes" in most human populations.

The Pima Indians of the American Southwest, the Eskimos, and the Australian aborigines are examples of populations where severe food shortages were once common occurrences. Today, when these people adopt a Western lifestyle, with bountiful food supplies, the very same "fat genes" that once increased their chances of survival are now manifesting themselves in obesity and its negative health consequences. Now that the Pima Indians have become "Westernized," they have the highest incidence of age-onset (Type II) diabetes of any population group.

Among Australian aborigines who have abandoned their traditional hunting and gathering lifestyle, a large percentage have become obese and developed "Western" diseases such as diabetes, high blood pressure, certain cancers, and clogged arteries. Australian physicians paid a group of these native Australians to return to the outback and the hunter-gatherer ways of their forebears. For the three-month study, all were taken off the drugs that had been prescribed for their diabetes and/or high blood pressure.

At the end of the study, both blood sugar and blood pressure had returned to normal levels in the subjects. The native diet, which was low in fat and high in fiber, along with increased activity, also produced significant weight loss.

At the end of the study, the aborigines opted to return to their previous lifestyle, and again they became obese, diabetic, and hypertensive. The "good" life had struck again.

By contrast, the islanders of the South Pacific generally had a fairly reliable food supply year-round. Despite the intrusion of Western culture and its high-fat diet into their tropical home, these people have remained fairly lean. It would appear that there are few individuals in these islands with an inherited predisposition to become fat.

METABOLIC DEFECTS ARE RARELY A CAUSE OF OBESITY

Precisely how "fat genes" enhance our ability to store fat has not been entirely worked out. Researchers have identified several inherited metabolic defects found in the fatty Zucker rat and the ob/ob mouse that invariably result in chubby little varmints. In the case of the fatty Zucker rat, even food restriction fails to alter body composition. You simply get fat little rodents instead of big fat rodents when you put these rats on a low-calorie diet. These metabolic defects are also associated with a number of other physiological disturbances ranging from diabetes and elevated blood lipids to poor resistance to cold. As we shall see, this inability to adapt to cold may underlie a primary defect in the metabolic "furnace" needed to burn stored fat.

However, serious metabolic defects, such as those found in genetically fat strains of mice and rats, may underlie some cases of extreme obesity in humans but are probably not present in most people who are less than 100 pounds overfat. If serious metabolic defects were the cause of most obesity, then obesity would be inevitable. Since the vast majority of people following a gorging lifestyle who switch to the L.A. Diet lose excess body fat and remain lean, most cases of obesity must be due to something besides "fat" genes.

FAT MAKES YOU FAT

The Japanese people are thought by many to be naturally lean. Less than 10 percent of middle-aged men and women are overweight by American standards. However, when they move to Hawaii or California and adopt a more Westernized diet, they quickly develop the same problems with weight control as most Westerners. In fact, the proliferation of American fast-food chains throughout Japan is making the average city dweller in Japan fatter each year.

The traditional Japanese diet is very low in fat by Western standards. As we shall see in Chapter 3, the low fat content of the traditional

Japanese diet is the main reason obesity is relatively uncommon in Japan.

So, the research summarized in this chapter should convince you that heredity is not destiny. Even if you seem to have inherited a tendency toward obesity, you *can* do something about it. The following chapters will show you that it's really fat, not your heritage, that makes you fat.

2
BODY FAT STORES: THE ROLE OF BODY TEMPERATURE REGULATION

The major conceptual breakthrough described in this book explains how a wide variety of environmental factors all impact directly or indirectly on body fat stores via their effect(s) on body temperature regulation. In simple terms, my theory states that *whatever warms you up slims you down.*

A CALORIE IS A MEASURE OF HEAT

One kilocalorie (aka *kcal* or *Calorie*) is the amount of heat needed to raise 1 kilogram (2.2 pounds) of water 1 degree centigrade (nearly 2 degrees Fahrenheit). One hundred calories is enough heat energy to bring a quart of ice water to a boil. That is a lot of heat. Most of the calories you consume each day are lost from the body as heat. Of the 100 calories you burn up walking a mile, 75 calories are released as heat within your body, and only 25 calories are actually converted into mechanical energy by your muscles.

Anyone who has ever kept a cold-blooded animal such as a frog, turtle, or snake for a pet is usually surprised by how little it needs to eat.

A small dog or cat will eat much more than a large snake of the same weight. This is because most of the food consumed is used to keep the dog's or cat's body warm.

To a certain extent, the less heat your body produces, the more insulation it needs. Subcutaneous fat (the fat layer under the skin), as we shall see, is a form of insulation. The less heat your body produces, the more insulation it needs to maintain a constant body temperature.

THE HYPOTHALAMUS REGULATES BODY TEMPERATURE AND APPETITE

Both body temperature and hunger are regulated by the same specialized area of the brain known as the *hypothalamus*. The hypothalamus detects body temperature through sensory cells within the skin and within the hypothalamus itself; these cells monitor the temperature of blood flowing through the brain. Figure 2.1 depicts the body as a house (1) and the temperature-sensing and regulating mechanism in the hypothalamus as a thermostat (2). The body's "thermostat" is set at 98.6 degrees Fahrenheit.

FIGURE 2.1

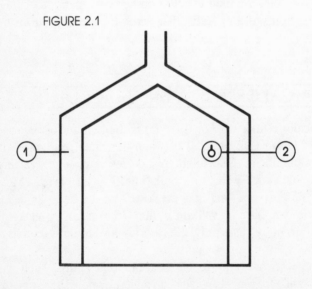

FIGURE 2.2

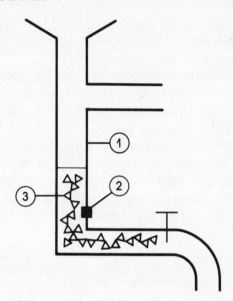

Other specialized cells within the hypothalamus monitor blood sugar levels and hormones associated with the regulation of blood sugar (e.g., insulin). In Figure 2.2, the body's storage capacity for carbohydrate is depicted as a fuel "storage tank" (1). The mechanism within the hypothalamus that detects the level of fuel (glycogen) stored within this tank is depicted as a "fuel gauge" (2). Glycogen, which is made up of chains of glucose (blood sugar) molecules, is depicted as chains of triangles within the fuel (carbohydrate) "storage tank" (3).

When the body runs low on stored carbohydrate (glycogen), its capacity to produce heat is compromised. When this happens, you feel hungry. Eating, as we shall see, warms you up. However, if you do not eat, or if you consciously restrict the amount you eat, you will begin to chill more easily, because your metabolic rate is slowing down. In the short run, your body can adapt by producing stress hormones that speed up the metabolic rate, but eventually you become cold, fatigued, depressed, and lethargic.

The body has a rather limited capacity to store carbohydrates. On a typical Western diet, about 1,000–1,800 calories of carbohydrate (as glycogen) can be stored, depending on body size. Much of this is in the muscles and not readily available to replenish a depleted blood sugar level. About 300–500 calories of glycogen are stored in the liver. From the liver, glycogen can be quickly mobilized to maintain blood sugar levels (fuel supply) between meals. When blood sugar levels drop, due to depletion of liver glycogen, you feel hungry.

When your skin temperature and/or blood temperature drops, you feel cold; this, like depletion of the glycogen stores, signals the hypothalamus that your body needs more fuel. Your hypothalamus signals you to increase your fuel supply by making you hungry. When you eat, you refill your depleted glycogen stores. After eating, the increased fuel supply temporarily speeds up your metabolic rate, which warms you up.

Body temperature regulation is critical to our survival as warm-blooded animals (homeotherms). In order to maintain a constant body temperature, we must carefully regulate the rate at which we burn calories.

Body Fat Is a Form of Insulation

The need to regulate body temperature explains why most warm-blooded animals are insulated. In the case of humans, we call that insulation subcutaneous (under the skin) fat.

One of the main functions of subcutaneous body fat is to hold heat in the body. This is why thin people often chill more easily and overfat people often perspire more easily than thin individuals when they exercise. Exercise dramatically increases heat production, which is one reason it helps to slim you down. (More on this in Chapter 4.)

BODY TEMPERATURE REGULATION

It should be obvious that increased insulation is one way of dealing with the stress of cold. Let's take a closer look at how we regulate our body temperature and then see how what we eat can affect the amount of body fat we store.

When we are hot, we sweat. As the sweat evaporates from our skin it cools the skin and the blood flowing near the skin. Panting serves the same function in dogs and cats. The brain also tells our muscles to relax when we are hot, and this reduces the amount of metabolic heat produced by the muscles. (This is why heat applied to stiff muscles tends to relax them.) Conversely, as we become cold the brain increases muscle tension, which burns more calories and tends to warm us up. If we continue to feel cold, we start to shiver, which produces even more heat.

The hypothalamus regulates body temperature. It appears that one of the ways it does so is by increasing or decreasing appetite.

It is much more important for a warm-blooded animal to regulate its body temperature than its body weight. An increase or decrease in body temperature of about 10 degrees or more is usually fatal, while gaining or losing 10 pounds of body fat is relatively inconsequential as far as survival is concerned.

When You Are Hot, You Lose Your Appetite

We have known for years that you lose your appetite when you run a fever. We have also known that working up a good sweat will also kill your appetite. Whatever warms you up slims you down.

Remember that food contains calories (stored heat energy) in the form of fat, protein, and carbohydrates. When the chemical bonds holding these molecules together are broken, energy is released. Some of this heat energy found in food is released during digestion, absorption, and storage. This is known as the *specific dynamic effect* or *specific dynamic action* of a meal. Eating with a fever or after exercise would only increase body temperature more due to the specific dynamic effect. This would increase the heat stress on the body. Therefore, your "intuition"—actually your hypothalamus at work—tells you to "starve a fever."

As we shall see, this specific dynamic effect varies considerably among various food components. This is one of the reasons why some food components are "fattening" and others are not. The kind of food you eat—in terms of its fat and carbohydrate content—is one of the most critical factors in determining how much body fat you will store.

Being Cold Heats Up Your Appetite

Scientific research has shown that animals placed in a cold environment eat much more food, doubling or even tripling their food intake. Despite enormous appetites, they do not gain weight, so it is clear that all of the food they consume is being used to regulate body temperature. Under extreme environmental conditions it becomes clear that one of the primary determinants of hunger is the need for a source of fuel to stoke the "metabolic furnace" and keep the homeotherm's blood warm.

It has been known for many years that people tend to gain a few pounds in the winter and lose them in the summer. Of course, now we compensate for variations in weather conditions primarily by wearing warmer clothes and staying indoors in the winter. In the summer, we turn on the air-conditioning. This means the amount of heat or cold stress most people experience nowadays is much too small to have any major impact on appetite or body fat regulation. Nevertheless, researchers have found that most people gain a few pounds in the winter and shed them again in the summer. Of course, some of this may be due to an increased consumption of fruits and salads in the summer months.

Fat as Insulation

As we have seen, one of the primary challenges faced by all warm-blooded animals is maintaining a constant body temperature. Figue 2.3 illustrates how body fat can keep you warm by acting as a fuel source for your metabolic furnace and by insulating you as subcutaneous fat.

The "storage tank" for fat in your body (1) has an unlimited capacity. A few individuals actually have over a million calories stored as fat. This fat is stored as triglyceride, which is indicated in Figure 2.3 as three circles because it is made up of three fatty acids. This fat or triglyceride is stored primarily in specialized cells throughout the body known as *adipocytes* (fat cells). Adipose tissue is simply a large group of fat cells.

The amount of fat stored in your body can be increased by increasing the amount of fat per cell (hypertrophy) or by increasing the number of fat cells (hyperplasia). In Figure 2.3, hypertrophy may increase the level within the storage tank, whereas hyperplasia may make the fat storage tank bigger.

In order to get out of the fat cells (storage tank) and into the bloodstream (2), the triglyceride or fat molecules must be broken down into single or free fatty acids (FFA). There are enzymes and hormones that regulate the release of FFA from the fat cells, and they are represented by the "output control valve" (3).

As fat cells get larger, they produce more enzymes that break triglycerides into free fatty acids. Therefore, in general, bigger cells release FFA

FIGURE 2.3

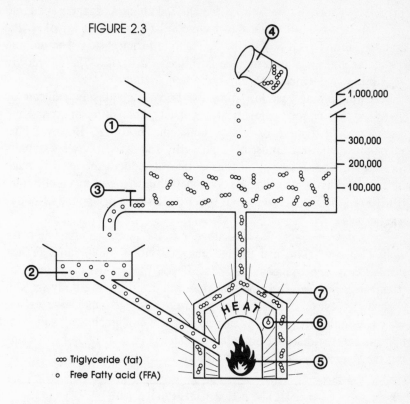

1,000,000

300,000

200,000

100,000

∞ Triglyceride (fat)
o Free Fatty acid (FFA)

more rapidly, which increases the metabolic rate. The same total amount of fat stored in twice as many cells would result in less FFA release and a slower metabolic rate, which is why hyperplastic obesity is associated with slower and more difficult weight loss than hypertrophic obesity.

As people become more obese, first cell size increases, but eventually the number of cells increases, which means very obese people have bigger storage tanks, and their fat set point is permanently elevated. No diet, including this one, can decrease the number of fat cells. Therefore, to the extent you have increased your fat cell number (increasing the size of the storage tank), you will be unable to completely lose all the fat you have gained. This may be somewhat discouraging to very obese people. Of course, switching to the L.A. Diet will reduce the level in the storage tank, so whether you have hypertrophic or hyperplastic obesity, you will still lose excess body fat.

When you are at a stable body weight, the amount of fat dumped into your fat storage tank each day from food (4) must be equal to the amount burned each day in the "metabolic furnace" (5). The amount burned in the metabolic furnace is influenced by the "thermostat" in your brain (6), which monitors body temperature.

The amount of heat lost from the body each day is reduced by increased "insulation" (7) (subcutaneous fat). Your skin can expand and contract to hold more or less subcutaneous body fat. However, that subcutaneous fat also must be kept warm. Increased body fat actually increases the need for calories faster than it reduces the need through insulation. This is why obese people have higher basal metabolic rates (BMRs) in the absolute sense but lower BMRs on a per-pound-of-body-weight basis.

The house in Figure 2.3 is analogous to the human body. The outer wall, like your skin, can expand and contract to hold more or less insulation or subcutaneous body fat. If you picture the outer walls as stretchable, you can imagine that the layer of insulating body fat will expand as the level of fat (triglyceride) in the storage tank above it rises. This is exactly what happens in your body. The "pinch test" and skin-fold calipers estimate the amount of fat stored in your body by measuring the layer of insulating body fat attached to your skin.

Sticky Fat and Deadly Fat

People vary somewhat in the percentage of their total body fat stored under their skin (as opposed to intra-abdominal fat around the organs). They also vary somewhat in terms of the location under their skin where fat is stored. For example, women tend to store more of their fat under the skin in the thighs and buttocks, whereas men tend to store more fat in the abdomen and upper torso. Recent research has shown that the abdominal fat releases FFA into the bloodstream much more readily than fat stored in the thighs and buttocks, especially when stimulated by hormones released during exercise and stress.

The difference in the ability to mobilize fat from these different locations is a real good news–bad news situation. The good news is that the fat located in your abdomen is much more easily mobilized by exercise than fat below the waist and thus is easier to get rid of. The bad news is that stress hormones (such as norepinephrine) will mobilize this fat, releasing excessive amounts of FFA into your bloodstream when they are not needed. These fatty acids, directly or indirectly, play havoc with your metabolism. There is growing evidence that both men and women with large stores of abdominal fat are much more likely to develop diabetes and cardiovascular disease.

In fact, women who have a waist-to-hip ratio of 0.8 or greater are eight times more likely to develop diabetes than women with the same amount of fat but with a greater portion located below their waist. There is growing evidence that men with a waist measurement as large as or larger than their hips are at very high risk for developing heart disease.

So the good news, if your body fat is primarily in the hips and thighs, is that it poses much less risk to your health and longevity. The bad news is that it is much tougher to get rid of. The only time this fat is readily mobilized is during breast-feeding. It appears that the fat located in the hips and buttocks region was nature's way of assuring an adequate supply of milk for the newborn.

In the long run, it really does us no good and a lot of harm to try to be what we are not. Nature designed us to graze, not gorge, and to breast-feed, not bottlefeed. Going against our biological heritage usually results in psychological and/or physical health problems. The L.A. Diet Program is the first permanent weight loss plan based on a scientific understanding of why we get fat and how we can become our leanest. It works because it is natural.

UNNATURAL WAYS TO LOSE WEIGHT

I suspect that one of the reasons cigarette smoking has remained so popular, particularly among young women, is that it artificially lowers the body's set point for body fat. An excellent review article on the effects of smoking on body fat storage by Drs. Jeffery Wack and Judith Rodin at Yale University was published in the February 1982 issue of *The American Journal of Clinical Nutrition.* They reviewed the scientific research that shows that smoking lowers insulin levels and increases the rate at which FFA are released from the fat cells. Increased FFA going to the metabolic furnace means increased heat production and decreased fat storage. This is one reason why smoking lowers the body's set point for body fat.

Smoking opens the output control valve (see Figure 2.3) from the fat storage tank, which artificially changes the ratio of fat to carbohydrate burned in the body's metabolic furnace. As we shall see in the next chapter, altering this fuel mix will alter the amount of fat stored in the body.

However, even though smoking can artificially lower your body's set point for stored fat, it is unnatural and unhealthy. On the average, smoking will lower your set point by 10 to 20 pounds, but you would have to gain at least 50 to 80 pounds of body fat to reduce your life expectancy as much as smoking a pack of cigarettes daily. In this case, the "cure" is clearly worse than the disease.

It should be noted that all drugs that lower the body's set point for body fat have only a temporary effect. Nicotine and diet pills (amphetamine derivatives) appear to act via the sympathetic nervous system to increase the release of FFA from the fat cells. Epinephrine (adrenaline) and norepinephrine are the primary hormones released by the action of the sympathetic nervous system. Epinephrine attaches to beta-receptors on the fat cells. This opens the output control valve of the fat storage tank shown in Figure 2.3. Drugs that block the effects of the sympathetic nervous system (called *beta-blockers*) usually slow the metabolic rate and cause people taking them to gain weight.

As soon as you stop taking diet pills, your body's set point for body fat will go right back where it was, and you'll eventually regain all the weight you lost. All of these drugs have been shown to have serious and even life-threatening side effects. Given the scientific evidence, it is hard to believe anyone but a charlatan would claim that diet pills are anything more than an expensive and often dangerous hoax.

DIETARY FAT BECOMES BODY FAT

No matter where the fat on your body is located, it all came from the same source—dietary fat. Research has shown that the composition of the fat in your body is almost identical to the composition of the fat in your diet. Seals eat fish, and their fat is similar to fish fat. The Greeks eat tons of olive oil, and their body fat is much more similar to olive oil than that of the Finns, who eat a lot of dairy products and have much harder (more saturated) fat. The Finns also have a higher incidence of hardening of their arteries because of this hard or saturated fat.

In the next chapter you will see why the fat you eat is the same fat that ends up on your hips, your thighs, your stomach, the backs of your arms, and under your chin. It is dietary fat that makes you fat. Regardless of where your fat is, the L.A. Diet is your best hope for losing the excess poundage and keeping it off.

3
FAT MAKES YOU FAT

Now that we have seen how important it is to maintain a nearly constant body temperature despite wide variations in environmental temperature and/or caloric intake, we will examine how the fuel mix in your diet— the ratio of fat to carbohydrate—affects heat production and fat storage.

In order to maintain a constant body temperature with a variable fuel source, it is necessary to store the fuel. If you put 10 logs in your fireplace at once, the fire will get too hot and overheat the room. A few hours later, when all the wood is burned up, the room will become too cold. In much the same way, your body would overheat if it burned up all the calories in a large meal as quickly as they were digested and absorbed, and you would become very cold at night. Thus, storing carbohydrates and fats is the key to maintaining a nearly constant body temperature.

Body fuel (energy or calories) is stored primarily as glycogen and fat in animals. As we have seen, the storage tank for fat (triglyceride) is much larger than that for carbohydrate (glycogen). This has important implications for regulating metabolic heat production, body temperature, and the desire to eat.

THE HEAT IN WHAT YOU EAT

The human body is mostly water (unless you are extremely obese, in which case your body's fat content can exceed its water content), so the error in assuming the heat capacity of the human body is the same as that of water is small enough to ignore for our purposes. With this assumption it is easy to estimate the change in body temperature that would occur if the entire caloric content of a meal were liberated immediately.

Let's calculate the rise in body temperature that a 110-pound (50-kilogram) woman would experience if all the heat in a 500-calorie meal were released instantly. If one calorie raises one kilogram of water one degree centigrade, then 500 calories would raise 50 kilograms 10 degrees centigrade or 18 degrees Fahrenheit (500 calories ÷ 50 kilograms = 10 degrees centigrade). This would elevate her body temperature from 98.6 to 116.6 degrees, which would be fatal.

Of course this can never happen because there are plenty of built-in biochemical and physiological mechanisms to prevent it. Even though most of the calories found in food are not liberated during digestion, absorption, and storage, some are. This amount is determined by the varying ability of the body to store fat, protein, and carbohydrate.

DIETARY-INDUCED THERMOGENESIS

The amount of heat released from fats and oils after a meal is relatively small compared to that released from carbohydrates and proteins. (This does not mean, however, that we are advocating a high-protein diet. For more information on the protein myth, see Chapter 6.) In other words, a meal high in carbohydrate and low in fat is more heat-producing (thermogenic) than one high in fat and low in carbohydrate. As mentioned earlier, the heat produced by eating is referred to as the *specific dynamic action (SDA)* or *specific dynamic effect* of food. It is also called the *heat increment,* which refers to the extra increment of heat produced above the resting metabolic rate or basal metabolic rate. This dietary-induced thermogenesis or heat production is one of the keys to understanding why fat makes you fat and why whatever warms you up slims you down.

Fat Has a Much Higher
Octane Rating Than Carbohydrate

Dietary-induced thermogenesis is largely the result of our body's differential ability to store fat and carbohydrate. Ounce for ounce, fats and oils have over twice the stored energy of sugars and starches (both carbohydrates). One gram of fat has about nine calories, compared to about four calories for a gram of carbohydrate. Since fats supply much more energy per ounce than carbohydrates, they have a higher octane rating.

In addition to being a low-octane fuel, carbohydrates stored in the body absorb a lot of water. In our bodies carbohydrates will contain about three parts of water for every part of starch (glycogen). When fully cooked, oatmeal, pasta, rice, and other starchy foods absorb about three times their original weight in water. One pound of carbohydrate stored as glycogen, with three times its weight in trapped water, would supply about 1 calorie per gram or only 454 calories per pound (1 pound equals 454 grams).

Since most animals move around a lot, it is very important that they not lug around a lot of low-octane fuel to run their metabolic "motors." Imagine the problems that would arise if the gas tank in your car had to be nine times larger in order to hold the same amount of fuel.

Fats and oils do not mix with water and can be stored in the cell without any appreciable need for extra water. This means that one pound of stored fat in your body contains approximately 4,000 calories (454 grams $\times$ 9 calories/gram = 4,086 calories). Since fat cells do contain a small amount of water, most nutritionists estimate that about 3,500 calories represent one pound of fatty tissue.

An average-weight American man (150 pounds) carries around about 120,000 calories as fat. This represents about 30 pounds. If all of this energy were stored instead as glycogen, the same amount of fuel energy would weigh 270 pounds. A 150-pound man with 30 pounds of fat would become a 390-pound man if all the energy stored in his body fat were stored instead as glycogen. Obviously, this would be impractical, and it is the main reason that animals that eat plants high in carbohydrates and low in fat preferentially store the fat and burn up the carbohydrates for energy, storing relatively little energy as glycogen (carbohydrate).

HOW DIET COMPOSITION AFFECTS BODY COMPOSITION

The human body's capacity to store carbohydrates is limited to under two pounds. At most, about 3,000 calories can be stored as glycogen. Nevertheless, it is very important that this small reserve not be depleted. Glycogen, stored in the liver, is the primary source of blood sugar between meals. Under normal circumstances the brain uses only blood sugar as its energy source. Without glycogen, however, your body is forced to break down proteins in order to prevent blood sugar levels from dropping too low. Just as the intelligent person would rather go out and chop or purchase more firewood rather than burn up his furniture to fuel the furnace, so does our body "prefer" to replenish its limited glycogen stores rather than break down the structural materials of its cells (proteins).

Glycogen, unlike fat, can be used to produce energy in the absence of oxygen. It is this process—known as *glycolysis*—that allows us to sprint, lift weights, or engage temporarily in any anaerobic activity. Anaerobic exercise, such as being able to run very fast and climb trees or hurl heavy rocks, undoubtedly contributed to the survival of our distant ancestors, so you can see why it was critical to our species survival. This is why the body carefully controls the amount of glycogen it has stored.

Maintaining glycogen stores within a fairly narrow range is just as important to us as maintaining our body temperature within a very narrow range. Too much or too little glycogen simply has such detrimental effects on our survival capacity that evolution "developed" a very sensitive feedback system to prevent this from happening. This feedback mechanism is depicted in Figure 3.1.

Figure 3.1 depicts the storage tank for carbohydrates (as glycogen) (1). We can see that about 1,800 calories are stored as glycogen (2). When the glycogen stores drop, this drop is detected by the fuel level sensor (3). How this sensor works is not entirely clear, but undoubtedly it involves a drop in the amount of blood sugar and/or hormonal changes associated with a dropping blood sugar level such as low insulin levels. When this happens, we feel hungry and must eat to replenish our glycogen stores.

In Figure 3.1 we can also see that there is an upper limit to the storage tank for glycogen. Under no circumstances can it hold more than 3,000

FIGURE 3.1

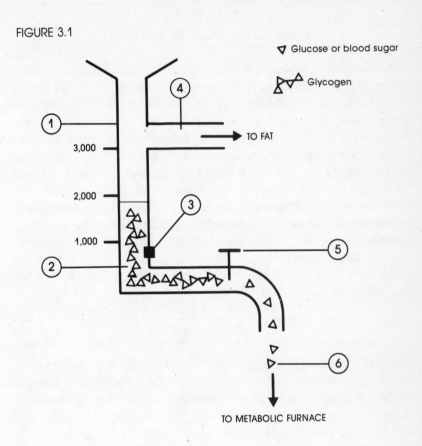

calories. When carbohydrate intake exceeds storage capacity, carbohydrates "flow" through the "overflow line" (4) and end up being converted into fat. However, this mechanism is rarely used by the body because about a fourth of the energy (calories) contained in the carbohydrate molecules is lost as heat in the conversion process. The extra heat released when carbohydrates are converted to fats over a short period of time quickly raises your body temperature, suppressing your appetite. This keeps you from overeating high-carbohydrate meals.

Glycogen Level in Tank
Determines Rate of Burning

The rate at which glycogen flows out of the storage tank is determined by the level of glycogen in it. The output control valve (5) can also be opened to allow more glucose to run into the metabolic furnace (6). The storage tank, in a sense, is like a coffee machine or bottled water dispenser. When the spout is open, the force of gravity pushes out more coffee or water when the dispenser is full than when it is nearly empty. This is exactly the way the storage tank for glycogen works in your body. And just as a high level of glycogen stored increases the flow of glucose molecules to the metabolic furnace, a low level of stored glycogen decreases the rate of carbohydrate burning. Since the metabolic furnace needs a more or less constant supply of fuel if it is to maintain a constant body temperature, the metabolic furnace must have another source of fuel to fall back on when glycogen stores are low. This alternative fuel source is fat.

Fat Storage

Figure 3.2 depicts fat storage in the body. In many ways fat storage is analogous to carbohydrate storage, but there are a few major differences.

The most obvious difference between fat and carbohydrate storage in the body is the size of the storage tanks. The average American has over 100 times as many calories stored as fat (triglyceride) as is stored as carbohydrate (glycogen). In this diagram we can see that 180,000 calories are stored as triglyceride (1). This would correspond to about 45 pounds of body fat. The 1,800 calories stored as glycogen depicted in Figure 3.1 would correspond to a body weight of 4 pounds.

Another important difference between carbohydrate storage and fat storage is that the storage tank for fat (2) has no overflow line to limit the amount of fat that can be stored. In the figure the upper limit of the tank is depicted as 1,000,000 calories of fat, which would weight just less than 250 pounds. This is the amount of body fat we would expect to find in a 450-pound individual (a 450-pound man would usually be 50 to 60 percent fat and 40 to 50 percent lean weight according to body composition analysis). People weighing more than that do exist, so the 1,000,000-calorie storage capacity can be exceeded. The key point to be

FIGURE 3.2

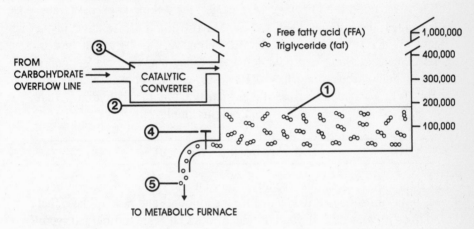

made here is that while there is a limit to the amount of carbohydrate the body can store, there is no limit when it comes to tucking away extra calories as fat.

Fats Can't Be Converted to Carbohydrates

Another difference is the "catalytic converter" (3), which converts any carbohydrates in the overflow line into fat and "pumps" them into the fat storage tank as triglyceride. It is important to note that this is a one-way mechanism; the body has no way of converting excess fat into carbohydrates. Therefore, diets higher in fat and lower in carbohydrate are less satisfying in the long run because you require a lot more total calories from such a diet to replenish your glycogen stores.

Fat Makes You Fat— Carbohydrates Only Make You Feel Guilty

As we have seen, the two primary triggers for eating are (1) to maintain the glycogen stores for quick energy bursts and (2) to provide sufficient heat to maintain body temperature. This is why there is relatively little to worry about from high-carbohydrate foods, *provided fat intake is kept very low.*

Starting in the mid-1950s, Americans were bombarded with diet books all condemning high-carbohydrate foods as the bane of dieters. These included the Drinking Man's Diet, the Atkins Diet, the Grapefruit Diet, the Stillman Diet, and the Mayo Clinic Diet, to name just a few. As a result, Americans started feeling very guilty about breads, pasta, cereals, fruits, and potatoes. Even today many people feel guilty about high-carbohydrate foods. However, as this book explains, this guilt is unwarranted because it is primarily fat, not carbohydrates, that ends up as the "love handles" and bulging thighs.

You Are What You Eat

It should be obvious that the amount of fat and carbohydrate you burn each day must be nearly identical to the amounts and ratio of these fuel sources in your diet. If you consumed more fat than you burned, your body fat stores would increase and you'd be gaining weight. Since body weight and body composition stay fairly constant over time, it is clear that your body must be burning fats and carbohydrates in the same proportion that they are found in your diet.

The ratio of fat to carbohydrate in your diet is one of the major determining factors for the ratio of fat to carbohydrate stored in your body. The old adage "you are what you eat" has an element of truth.

How Dietary Fat Makes You Fat

In Figure 3.3, we can see our subject has 1,800 calories stored as glycogen and 180,000 calories stored as fat. Above the storage tanks is a "cylinder" (1). This cylinder depicts the average amount of fat and carbohydrate consumed in a day by a typical middle-aged man. On a typical day, he would consume about 1,000 calories each of fat and carbohydrate (and another 400 calories as protein, which we'll ignore for the time being).

The contents of this cylinder are separated after being absorbed into the body into "measuring cups" (1). In this case, we can see that each measuring cup has 1,000 calories of either fat or carbohydrate. This 50:50 ratio of fat to carbohydrate is the norm for Americans and affluent Europeans.

Figure 3.3 shows the *level* of triglyceride and glycogen in their respective storage tanks is the same even though the fat storage tank holds 100 times as much total energy (calories) (2). However, it is the *level* and not the absolute amount of fuel in each storage tank that determines the rate at which FFA and glucose flow out of storage and into the bloodstream (3) on their way to the metabolic furnace (4), where they are burned ultimately to produce heat. This is, perhaps, the most important point to grasp from this model.

FIGURE 3.3

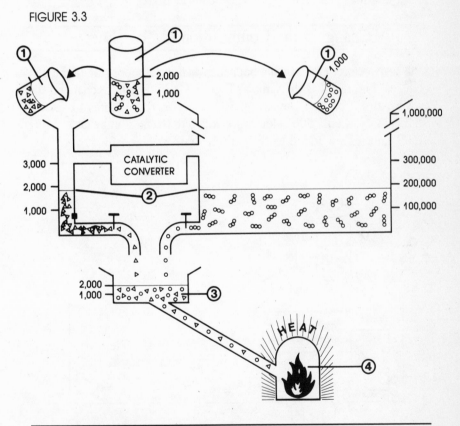

Fuel Level Determines Rate of Burning

In our analogy, if the level of fuel in either tank doubled, twice as much fuel would flow from that storage tank. If the level of fuel in one storage tank dropped very low, only a trickle would flow through the output control valve and into the metabolic furnace. Unless the level of fuel in the other storage tank were simultaneously increased, there would be less total fuel available for the metabolic furnace. This would result in a slowdown of the metabolic rate and less heat production.

If this happened, your body temperature would start to drop, which would make you hungry. A drop in stored carbohydrate (glycogen) would be detected by the fuel level sensor, and this also makes you hungry. It may even make you crave carbohydrates.

Changing the Composition of Your Diet

Let's take a closer look at what happens when the composition of the diet changes. Figure 3.4 is the same as Figure 3.3, but we have changed the fuel mixture from the typical 50:50 ratio of carbohydrates to fats to 75:25 (1). Now only 500 calories are added to the fat storage tank, while 1,500 calories are added to the carbohydrate storage tank (1).

FIGURE 3.4

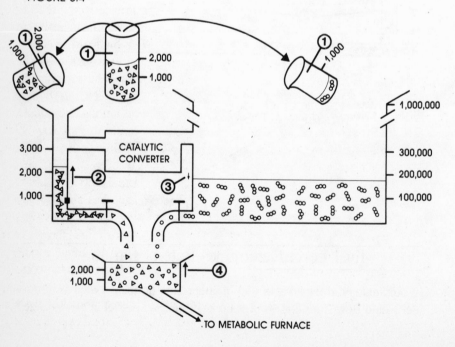

You can see that an extra 500 calories of carbohydrate—an increase from 1,800 to 2,300 calories—will raise the level of glycogen in the carbohydrate storage tank (2) by 28 percent. However, adding 500 calories instead of 1,000 calories to the fat storage tank reduces the amount of fat stored (3) from 180,000 to 179,500 calories, much less than a 0.3 percent drop.

Therefore, the rate at which carbohydrates are released into the metabolic furnace has increased by 28 percent. By the end of the day, an extra 500 calories of glucose pass through the output control valve of the carbohydrate storage tank and into the bloodstream on their way to the metabolic furnace. However, since 500 fewer calories entering the fat storage tank had no significant effect on the level of fat stored in the body, the release of FFA from the fat storage tank is hardly affected (3). As a result, the rate of FFA release is decreased by no more than 1 or 2 calories. This is why the total amount of metabolic fuel released from storage is increased by nearly 500 calories (4) even though there was no net increase in calorie intake. *This is why high-carbohydrate, low-fat meals increase heat production and high-fat, low-carbohydrate meals slow it down.*

An extra 500 calories going to the metabolic furnace would tend to warm you up, which means we would expect a significant drop in appetite and a reduction in food intake. As long as a high-carbohydrate, low-fat diet is consumed, this reduction in food intake will continue until a new equilibrium is reached and the mix of fuels entering the metabolic furnace is again in equilibrium with the diet. (Precisely how long it will take to reach a new set point for fat varies among individuals; for information on what to expect, see the last chapter in Part I.)

Figure 3.5 shows the new equilibration point where the level of fat stored is now three times lower than the level of glycogen stored (2 and 3). Our subject's body fat stores have dropped from 180,000 to about 70,000 calories (2). Since each pound of fatty tissue has about 3,500 calories, a drop of 110,000 calories in the fat storage tank would correspond to a 31.5-pound weight loss. By contrast, the extra 500 calories in the carbohydrate storage tank (3) would correspond to about a one-pound weight gain. As a result, our subject's total body weight would eventually drop by over 30 pounds.

Since it takes about 15 calories a day to keep each pound of body tissue warm (at 98.6 degrees Fahrenheit), our subject's total caloric need

FIGURE 3.5

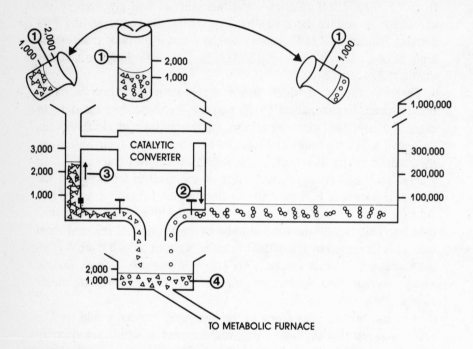

TO METABOLIC FURNACE

has dropped along with his weight. The drop in caloric need would predictably be about 450 calories. However, because some of this weight loss was insulating subcutaneous fat, his total caloric need would now be about 400 calories less per day. This is approximately the amount of fuel he would need to meet his new metabolic needs and keep his now smaller body warm.

In Figure 3.5 we can see that a total of 1,600 calories are now consumed daily (1). This is 400 calories fewer than before our subject reduced his fat stores. Of these, 1,600 calories, 1,200 come from carbohydrate and only 400 from fat. This is the same 75:25 ratio our subject has been consuming since switching from the 50:50 mix of the typical American diet. At 1,600 calories per day, our subject is once again burning the same amount and mix of metabolic fuel as he is consuming. The amount of fats and carbohydrates entering the bloodstream (4) on their way to the metabolic furnace is now the same as the ratio of fat to carbohydrate in his new low-fat, high-carbohydrate diet.

Now he has only 17 pounds of stored body fat instead of 45 pounds. Since he has lost about 30 pounds, he needs less food to stay warm. His metabolic rate has not dropped but actually *increased* slightly on a per-pound-of-body-weight basis because he has lost over half his insulating body fat.

If, instead of switching from a 50:50 mix of carbohydrate to fat to a 75:25 mix, our subject switched to a 25:75 mix of carbohydrate to fat, his level of body fat would double, and he would gain about 50 pounds. His total caloric intake from fat and carbohydrate would increase by nearly 700 calories per day.

Traditionally, it would have been argued that our subject gained the weight because he overate. In fact, he overeats because he gains the weight. His extra 50 pounds of body weight (mostly fat) still have to be kept warm. As mentioned previously, about 15 calories per day are required for each extra pound of body weight. This is why fat makes you fat and you are what you eat. The higher percentage of fat in your diet, the higher the percentage of fat stored in your body.

4

WARMING UP TO EXERCISE

Most people who need to lose weight are not thrilled by admonitions to exercise. Slogans like "no pain, no gain" scare off all but the hardiest and most determined. I am not going to tell you that exercise is not important; the scientific evidence proves otherwise. Indeed, a recent survey of 300 people who lost 70 pounds or more and kept it off found that the only two things that they all did were to reduce dietary fat and increase activity. The good news is that the exercise must be fun and moderate most of the time rather than painful and strenuous.

Strenuous exercise is exercise done at a heart rate above the training heart rate (discussed later in this chapter). Any exercise that cannot be maintained for 30 to 45 minutes should be considered too strenuous. In Figure 4.1 we can see why strenuous exercise can actually be counterproductive to fat loss. Our subject burned up more carbohydrate (glycogen) than fat during his strenuous workout (1). The hormones released during exercise open up the output control valves on both the fat and carbohydrate storage tanks (2). When aerobic exercise is strenuous, 70 to 90 percent of the calories burned are carbohydrate. This causes a big drop in the level of glycogen stored after one and a half hours, but only a small and insignificant drop in the level of triglyceride stored (3).

FIGURE 4.1

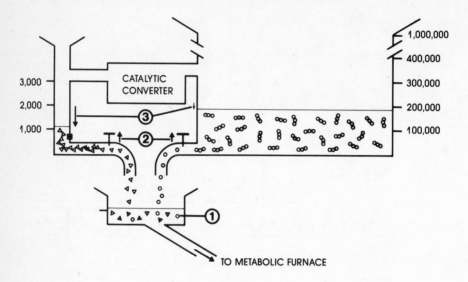

This big drop in stored glycogen would trigger the fuel sensor in the glycogen storage tank. As we have seen, depletion of stored carbohydrate makes us hungry. If the meal we consume is not at least 70 to 90 percent carbohydrate, the net result of strenuous exercise can be weight gain, not loss. This is especially true in unfit individuals. Aerobic training greatly increases the muscles' ability to burn fatty acids. Burning more fatty acids spares muscle and liver glycogen stores. When a relatively greater proportion of fat is burned, you feel less hungry after exercise than when you burn primarily carbohydrate.

THE COLD, HARD FACTS ON EXERCISE AND WEIGHT CONTROL

Before giving the cold shoulder to the notion of regular exercise, you need to understand all of the cold, hard facts. The most important one is that warming up slims you down. This chapter will help you warm up to the idea of exercising.

Other Health Benefits of Regular Exercise

Besides helping you lose weight, exercise has other benefits that can actually make your transition to the L.A. Diet lifestyle easier.

- First, and probably most important if you're discouraged by all the changes you'll have to make in your life, is that the reason most people who exercise regularly give for doing it is that it makes them feel better. Whether this is due to changes in neurotransmitter (e.g., endorphins) levels and/or better blood flow to the brain or simply the tension-releasing effects on muscles has not been adequately worked out, but that does not change the fact that you will almost certainly feel better in the long run if you exercise at least three or four times per week. Exercise also works as well as any medication for relieving mild depression.
- Exercise (unless overdone) is probably one of the most important factors for reducing the risk of osteoporosis.
- There is even mounting evidence that regular aerobic exercise can delay and even partially reverse some of the unpleasant effects we associate with growing old. A recent editorial in the *Annals of Internal Medicine* (November 1986, 783–785), entitled "Exercise and Aging," discusses these and other health benefits and estimates that regular exercise could add up to 10 years to your life expectancy.

People can give all sorts of excuses for not exercising regularly. The hardest part about exercise is starting. Once you've done it for a few months, you probably won't think much of the typical excuses ("not enough time" and "don't have the energy"). You simply will feel too good to stop.

How Exercise Contributes to Weight Loss

Exercise is the most effective way to stoke your metabolic furnace and heat up your body. Seventy-five percent of the calories you burn up while exercising are converted to heat, and only 25 percent actually end up being converted to mechanical energy to contract your muscles. That is why the right kind of exercise will warm you up and slim you down.

The epidemiological evidence from human populations and research on experimental animals supports the same theories about how diet and exercise interact to cause obesity in genetically susceptible individuals: (1) on a low-fat diet obesity will be relatively uncommon even in fairly sedentary populations; (2) the higher the percentage of calories from fat in the traditional diet of a given population, the greater the incidence of obesity; and (3) within a population consuming a high-fat diet, those who are the least active have the highest probability of becoming obese. The studies that follow provide strong evidence in support of these theories.

For the past 15-plus years Dr. Ancel Keys at the University of Minnesota has been studying various human populations in an attempt to better understand what factors contribute to a variety of diseases (especially cardiovascular disease). We can get some idea about how diet and exercise may affect a population by looking at populations with similar diets and different activity levels or with different diets and similar activity levels.

For example, as shown in Table 4.1, when Dr. Keys looked at two Yugoslavian communities with similar diets (Slavonia, 31.9 percent fat, and Zrejanin, 32.6 percent fat) but differing levels of customary activity, he found obesity much more prevalent in the much less active Zrejanin men (48 percent with a BMI greater than 25) than in the Slavonia men (28 percent with a BMI greater than 25). (BMI stands for *body mass index,* which is a measure of weight for height. Men with a BMI greater than 25 are considered to be overweight.)

Table 4.1 also contrasts U.S. railroad workers in Minnesota with men living in East Finland. Again the percentage of calories from fat in the

TABLE 4.1

Cohort	Dietary Fat % Calories	Activity Class (%)* 1	2	3	Obesity % BMI >25
Slavonia	31.9	17.1	9.2	73.7	28.0
Zrejanin	32.6	35.2	35.2	29.6	47.7
East Finland	38.5	9.6	12.6	73.8	25.1
U.S. Railroad**	38.0	49.7	35.3	0.0	56.5
Tanushimaru	9.0	3.9	36.6	59.5	9.1

*1 = sedentary; 2 = moderate activity; 3 = very active
**15% railroad workers' activity fell between classes 1 and 2

diets of the Americans and Finns is quite similar (38.0 vs. 38.5 percent). However, men in this Finnish community were much more active than the U.S. railroad workers, none of whom were classed as very active.

The human population with the lowest incidence of obesity was a Japanese community (Tanashimaru), most of whom were fairly active and consumed a low-fat diet (9 percent of total calories). Compared to the generally sedentary U.S. railroad employees, obesity in this Japanese community was more than six times less frequent (56.5 vs 9.1 percent).

In addition, obesity in Japanese cities where activity levels are generally in the sedentary classification is also uncommon by American standards. One study found that fewer than 10 percent of Japanese men aged 45 to 65 were overweight, while over 60 percent of a comparable group of American men were overweight. Since there is little difference in the activity of middle-aged Japanese and American men, the rarity of obesity in Japan cannot be attributed to differences in exercise.

When the Japanese move to Hawaii and California and begin consuming a more Westernized diet (higher in fat), the incidence of obesity becomes similar to that of Americans of European ancestry. This suggests that it is the fat content of the diet, rather than racial differences, that accounts for the low prevalence of obesity in countries like Japan, China, and Korea, where the typical diet is low in fat and high in carbohydrate. If the difference were racial or genetic, then we would not expect Asians consuming a high-fat diet to get fat.

Indeed, given an inherited tendency to store fat easily, obesity is all but inevitable for people who gorge on high-fat foods (most animal products, nuts, and refined fats and oils) and lead a sedentary lifestyle. Only those individuals who inherit either a relatively small fat storage tank and/or a relatively wide-open output control valve on this storage tank would remain fairly lean leading a sedentary lifestyle and consuming high-fat diet.

These theories are consistent with our theory that fat makes you fat and whatever warms you up slims you down. Exercise, as we shall see, is the most effective way to warm you up and burn off stored fat at the same time. The amount of heat produced by even modest exercise is sufficient to reduce your desire to eat. Let's take a look at the effects of exercise on the caloric output of human subjects and see how exercise fits into our model for understanding obesity.

Effect of Exercise on Spontaneous Caloric Intake

Dr. Rosy Woo and colleagues at Roosevelt Hospital Center and Columbia University studied the effects of mild and moderate exercise on the caloric balance of six obese women (ages 22 to 61) in a controlled hospital environment. The women were allowed to eat as much as they wanted to from fairly typical American fare. Everything they ate was carefully (but discreetly) monitored.

Each subject was allowed to choose her own exercise level on a treadmill with a slight uphill grade (2.5 percent). On the average they chose to walk at about a 3 mph pace. Table 4.2 shows the effects of mild (an extra 200 calories/day) and moderate (an extra 500 calories/day) exercise on overall energy (caloric) balance.

TABLE 4.2

	Activity Level		
	Sedentary	Mild	Moderate
Calories consumed	2,233	2,305	2,345
Calories burned	2,221	2,419	2,714
Balance	+11	−114	−369

Adapted from *American Journal of Clinical Nutrition*, 1982 (36:470–477).

We can see from the table that the subjects were in caloric balance when they were sedentary (+11 calories). However, even burning up an extra 200 calories per day put them into a negative calorie balance. Since it takes about 15 calories to keep each pound of body weight warm (or meet its metabolic needs), we can predict how much weight this negative caloric balance would translate into. In the long run this 114-calorie deficit would mean a weight loss of about 8 pounds. When these women exercised moderately (burned an extra 500 calories daily), the caloric difference grew to 369 calories, which ultimately would translate into a weight loss of 25 pounds.

The diet used in this study was not low in fat and high in carbohydrate. In addition, the women in this study certainly had a strong inherited predisposition to store fat. In terms of our model, they had a very large fat storage tank. Had they been consuming a high-carbohydrate diet, the effects of exercise would have been much greater because the exercise would be emptying the fat and carbohydrate storage tanks by approximately the same number of calories, but a relatively smaller amount of fat compared to carbohydrate in the L.A. Diet would have restored the glycogen reserves while allowing for a net deficit in the fat reserves.

With a "normal" diet, which is about a 50:50 mix of carbohydrate and fat, aerobic exercise brings little net loss of fat because replacing the glycogen stores to their former (pre-exercise) level necessitates replacing the fat as well. On the L.A. Diet this does not occur.

The authors of this study were not impressed by their results, concluding that " . . . the effects of exercise alone in the treatment of obesity will be tempered by the dietary milieu in which it is imposed." In other words, Dr. Woo and her colleagues felt that exercise alone gave unsatisfactory results for these women, who averaged over 200 pounds and needed to lose at least 50 to 100 pounds to reach their ideal body weight. Even with moderate exercise they could not have hoped to reach their ideal weight unless they also changed their diet.

The moral of this research is that for every mile you walk each day you can expect an eventual drop in body weight of about four to six pounds. (Women weighing about 200 pounds burn up about 100 calories for every mile they walk; since the women in the Woo study burned 200 calories and would lose eight pounds, we can predict that 100 calories burned would yield about half as much weight loss.) Since all healthy people ought to walk a minimum of three or four miles a day, exercise alone may be sufficent to keep you at your ideal body weight if you are only 10 to 20 pounds overweight. Again, this is not a green light for gorging. Adopting the L.A. Diet could prevent you from suffering the same fate as running enthusiast Jim Fixx, who kept his weight under control by running but paid the ultimate price for gorging—a heart attack while jogging.

HOW TO EXERCISE TO MAXIMIZE FAT BURNING

There is a lot of confusion about what type of exercise is best for burning off excess body fat. One group argues that the more strenuous the exercise, the more calories you burn, which ultimately means "harder is better." Another group argues that the more strenuous the exercise, the smaller the percentage of fat calories burned. The first group then argues that only strenuous exercise can increase your fitness level and that a higher fitness level increases your ability to burn fat. To which the second group responds that you can't keep up strenuous exercise long enough to burn much fat. As we shall see, there is some truth to all these arguments. The best way to exercise, from a scientific viewpoint, lies somewhere between these two schools of thought.

Much of this debate can be resolved by examining Figure 4.2. It shows the absolute amount and ratio of both fat and carbohydrates burned during one hour of exercise of increasing intensity.

You can see in Figure 4.2 that at rest our reference man burns about 90 calories per hour. Since he is consuming the typical American diet, the mix of carbohydrates to fats burned is 50:50 or in this case 45:45 since that is the ratio of these two fuel sources in his diet. If he walks two miles in an hour, he will burn an additional 200 calories. But the mix

FIGURE 4.2

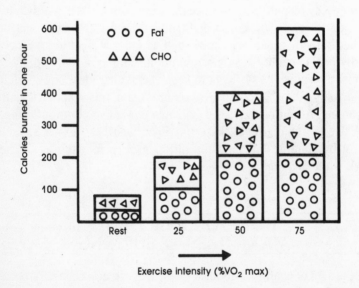

stays about the same, so he burns an extra 100 calories of both fat and carbohydrate. If he walks briskly (at 4 mph), he will burn up 400 calories, but the mix will still be about 50:50.

However, if he jogs at a moderate pace of 6 mph, he will burn no more fat than when he was walking briskly. Now he is burning twice as much carbohydrate as fat. At about 50 percent of your maximum work output, the output control valve on your fat storage tank is wide open and the maximum amount of FFA are pouring into your bloodstream to be burned for energy.

If you will recall our model for understanding obesity, you will remember that the carbohydrate storage tank usually contains fewer than 2,000 calories of stored glycogen. Burning up 600 calories of glycogen would put a significant dent in our subject's glycogen stores. This could set off the fuel level sensor, which would increase the desire to eat.

Furthermore, if the fuel mix consumed was a 50:50 mixture of carbohydrate to fat, we can see that moderate exercise would actually encourage the consumption of more fat than was lost during exercise since it would take 800 calories from a 50:50 mix to replace the 400 calories of glycogen burned up while running six miles. However, if a low-fat meal follows exercise, it will be possible to replace all of the 400 calories of glycogen and still be in a negative fat balance. This is why grazing and exercise are so effective for getting rid of excess body fat stores.

The only reason that moderate and intense exercise doesn't make people consuming a high-fat diet fat is that the tremendous amount of heat produced signals the brain (the hypothalamus) to eat less. You will recall that each calorie can raise one kilogram of water one degree centigrade. With exercise, 25 percent of the energy is converted into mechanical force by the muscles. The other 75 percent of the calories are released as heat, so we can calculate the amount of body heat produced during a six-mile run as follows:

$$600 \text{ cal} \times 0.75 = 450 \text{ cal released as heat (100 cal per mile)}$$
$$450 \text{ cal} \div 70 \text{ kg} = 6.4° \text{ centigrade or } 11.6° \text{ Fahrenheit}$$

Since this would raise our reference man's body temperature to over 110 degrees Fahrenheit, which would be fatal, he sweats. Sweating is your body's form of air-conditioning. However, whenever the air conditioner is turned on, the appetite is turned off. When the body consistently has trouble getting rid of excessive heat production, it also reduces its subcutaneous fat pads (insulation). This is why even moderately intense exercise can aid weight loss, provided it warms you up.

Prolonged Exercise Changes the Fuel Mix

Researchers have noted that the longer you exercise, the greater the proportion of fat to carbohydrate burned for energy. Since one of the goals of the L.A. Diet is to reduce the body's fat stores, it should be clear that the longer you exercise, the closer you will come to achieving your goal.

Why prolonged exercise burns more fat than carbohydrate is illustrated in Figures 4.3 and 4.4. In Figure 4.3 you can see that the levels of carbohydrate (glycogen) and fat (triglyceride) in their respective storage tanks are about equal when our subject starts to exercise (1). This means that initially the ratio of fat to carbohydrate flowing out of the storage tanks is a 50:50 mix (2).

Now, if you look at the situation after a two- to three-hour walk (Figure 4.4), you can see quite a difference. The storage tank for carbohydrates is so much smaller than the storage tank for fats that its fuel level drops much more rapidly. As you can see, the level of fuel stored as glycogen has dropped significantly after two to three hours of walking, but there is no significant change in the level of fuel stored as triglyceride (1). After all, burning up a few hundred calories of fat is not going to make a dent in the initial 180,000 calories stored. On the other hand, burning up a few hundred calories of carbohydrate will significantly deplete the stored glycogen.

Depletion of stored glycogen occurs more rapidly at higher intensity levels. In two to three hours a marathon runner can deplete his or her glycogen stores to the point where there is an inadequate fuel supply to maintain a fast pace. This is called "hitting the wall" and is the reason most endurance athletes carbohydrate-load before a big race. However, except for serious athletes, it is unrealistic to expect most individuals will deplete their glycogen stores with strenuous exercise.

In order to maintain the same amount of fuel for the muscles as the glycogen stores drop, your body releases epinephrine (adrenaline) and decreases its output of insulin. In our model these hormonal shifts are

FIGURE 4.3

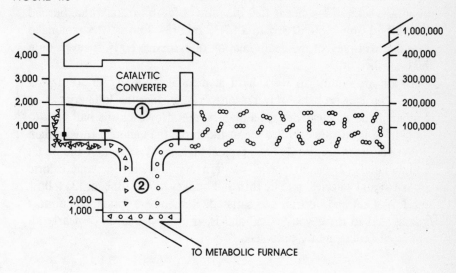

TO METABOLIC FURNACE

FIGURE 4.4

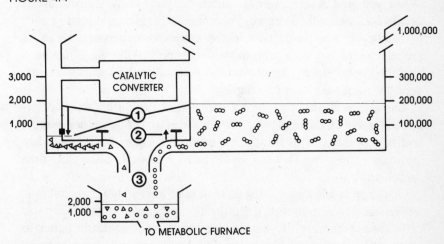

TO METABOLIC FURNACE

indicated by the opening of the output control valve on the fat storage tank (2). This means that free fatty acids will now flow more rapidly out of the fat storage tank even though the level in the reservoir remains about the same. This means that the ratio of fat to carbohydrate burned has shifted from a 50:50 mix to a 67:33 mix (3). This is why prolonged exercise will prevent the accumulation of excessive body fat even on a high-fat diet.

If you are willing to work hard at manual labor five or six days a week, you can probably stay reasonably lean, like the lumberjacks in Finland, who stay lean despite a high-fat diet. However, if a half hour to an hour of moderate exercise seems like more than enough to you, then you have three choices: (1) eat a typical high-fat Western diet and be fat and satiated, (2) eat a typical Western diet and restrict your caloric intake (count calories) and be thin and hungry all the time, or (3) follow the L.A. Diet and be lean and satiated. Remember, option 2 is almost guaranteed to drive you "nuts" and is, in fact, the cause of nearly all eating disorders, as we have seen.

GETTING THE MOST OUT OF YOUR EXERCISE

When you first wake up in the morning, your body temperature is usually well below 98.6 degrees Fahrenheit. This is due, at least in part, to a drop in heat production in the early morning hours, which is probably secondary to a drop in the fuel supply. After all, it has been about 10 hours since you refueled, so it should not be surprising that your glycogen stores are running low.

You will recall that the ratio of carbohydrate to fat burned is determined largely by the levels of glycogen and triglyceride in their respective storage tanks. This means that exercising before breakfast (when glycogen stores are lowest) will burn relatively more fat than carbohydrate.

On the other hand, exercising an hour or so after a high-carbohydrate, low-fat meal will minimize the utilization of stored fat and maximize carbohydrate burning. If you become too thin, it would be better to exercise after breakfast or in the evening. Nevertheless, how you exercise is much more important in determining body composition than the time of day.

If you can't bring yourself to exercise first thing in the morning, you can still benefit greatly from the right type of exercise.

Before we get into types of exercise, keep in mind that stretching is part of a total fitness plan. If you want to look and feel your best, stretching, like weight training, can be part of your total fitness program. The best time to stretch is after (not before) you warm yourself up with aerobic or long slow distance exercise. When your muscles, ligaments, and tendons are cold, they tear much more easily. When they are warmed up after a good workout, they become much more pliable. To get the greatest benefit from stretching you should not "bounce" (as you see people do in many health clubs and videos). Each stretch should be held 30 to 60 seconds.

Long Slow Distance

Most of the exercise you need to remain fit, trim, and healthy falls into the category of "long slow distance." For most people, this means brisk walking or a very comfortable pace on an exercise bike. Long slow distance exercise will warm you up without wearing you out. With this type of exercise your heart rate will be just below the lower end of the training heart rate range shown in Table 4.3. Build your mileage up slowly. If you try to do too much too soon, you will be more likely to injure yourself. Remember, you are building a lifelong healthy habit; you are not training for the Olympics.

TABLE 4.3

Age in Years	Maximum Heart Rate	Training Heart Rate
10	210	135–170
20	200	125–160
30	190	120–150
40	180	115–145
50	170	105–135
60	160	100–125

Over 60: increase heart rate 20–35 beats above resting level

Aeorbic Conditioning

Even though most of your exercise will fall into this long slow distance category, it is wise to do some aerobic conditioning as well to get the most out of this comfortable long slow distance training. Aerobic conditioning or training makes the output control valve on the fat storage tank open wider and more quickly in response to exercise. This means your body will burn free fatty acids more efficiently during more moderate exercise below the training heart rate. Burning FFA has a sparing effect on the glycogen stores. Since you eat to replenish your glycogen stores (there is no fuel level sensor on the fat storage tank), this will help you to lose body fat without increasing your appetite.

You will need to do about 20 to 30 minutes of aerobic conditioning three or four times per week. This means brisk walking, jogging, cycling, or riding an exercise bike at a pace that keeps your heart rate within the training range for your age, shown in Table 4.3.

The Training Effect

It is best to increase your pace gradually so that you get your heart rate up to the minimal training level in about five minutes (warm up). The minimal training level depends on your age. Table 4.3 shows the training heart rate by age. The minimal training heart rate is the low end of this range. Below this level there is little or no "training effect."

Above the training heart rate you start reaching a point of diminishing returns. The effort needed to maintain the faster pace increases rapidly, but the gains in fitness increase only slightly. So unless you wish to be competitive in 10Ks and marathons, it is pointless to push yourself that hard. Healthy exercise is not "punishment for dietary indiscretions" but a useful tool for losing excess body fat and feeling better.

Once you have increased your heart rate to the training range, you must keep it there for at least 20 minutes to get this training effect. After 20 to 50 minutes within this training heart range, it is best to gradually slow your pace for another five minutes before stopping (cool down). If you stay near the low end of this range, it is best to do at least 40 to 50 minutes at the training heart rate. Near the top of this range, 20 to 30 minutes is sufficient to get an adequate training effect.

The training effect is important for strengthening your heart and improving your overall fitness level. It will also improve your feeling of well-being. With a higher level of fitness you will be able to burn more fat with less effort.

Why Swimming Leaves You Fit and Fat

One of the great paradoxes in the weight control field concerns the ineffectiveness of swimming as an aid to weight loss. Until now there has been no convincing explanation of this paradox. After all, swimming, running, and cycling are equally effective for burning calories and are equally effective for improving your cardiovascular system. Why, then, should swimming be relatively ineffective in comparison with jogging or cycling for reducing body fat?

Covert Bailey was close to the answer when he made the following observation in *Fit or Fat?*:

> Swimming will get your heart and lungs in excellent aerobic condition. It's also great for limbering up all the muscles in the arms and legs. I do not recommend it, however, if you're overfat. There is no reduction in fat when a person embarks on a swimming program. This has been substantiated by body fat tests done in my clinic, Stanford University's water immersion testing program, and Dr. Ken Cooper's clinic in Texas.

Bailey continues:

> In contrast to the runner's body, which will shed as much weight as possible to provide more speed and agility, the swimmer's body tends to conserve its fat in order to provide warmth and buoyancy during exercise. Every sea-living mammal has made a similar adaption. Whales, seals, and otters have large amounts of fat covering very well trained muscles. In other words, swimming is a great aerobic exercise, but you'd better add some other exercise to your program if you're overfat.

Water has a high heat capacity compared to air. No one in his right mind would stick his hand into boiling water (212 degrees Fahrenheit). However, we think nothing of reaching into a 425-degree oven to pull out a baked potato. It is this difference in the capacity to hold heat that makes swimming a dangerous sport for dieters. You will recall that whatever warms you up slims you down. Well, swimming, even in tepid water, will drain so much heat out of your body that even vigorous swimming cannot maintain your body temperature.

At the same temperature, water will drain heat from your body 30 times faster than air. Even a very fit individual could increase his heat production only about 15-fold through vigorous exercise. This means he would be losing heat from his body much faster while swimming all-out than sitting quietly in the air. For less fit individuals this difference would be even greater. Prolonged, strenuous swimming workouts cool your body temperature and deplete your glycogen stores at the same time.

When you swim, particularly in cold water, you feel hungry afterward. This would not happen if aerobic exercise directly suppressed appetite. Exercise suppresses appetitie and causes a loss of insulating body fat *only if it warms you up*. Swimming, particularly in cold water, is counterproductive if you are trying to get rid of excess body fat. If it doesn't warm you up, it won't slim you down.

RISKS AND BENEFITS OF TRAINING

If you are older than 35 to 40 or have any questions about the risks of starting an exercise program, it is generally recommended that you check with your doctor before starting to train. Nevertheless, for the vast majority of people the dangers of inactivity greatly exceed the dangers of regular exercise, so most people would be better off training than waiting indefinitely to see their doctor before daring to start. This does not apply to people with advanced cardiovascular disease.

Dr. Per-Olof Astrand, the famous Swedish exercise physiologist, once said that "anyone contemplating an inactive lifestyle should have a thorough physical examination to see if his body can withstand it." The same could be said about anyone contemplating following a gorging diet. People who adopt the L.A. Diet will be much less likely in the long run to develop cardiovascular disease.

5

FINE-TUNING THE L.A. DIET

Now that we've seen how fat makes you fat and why anything that warms you up slims you down, it is time to do a little fine-tuning of the L.A. Diet.

The scientific, clinical, and epidemiological evidence all point to a high-fat diet and a sedentary lifestyle as the primary controllable risk factors leading to the accumulation of excessive body fat. As we saw in Chapter 1, an inherited tendency to store excess body fat is also involved. However, for most people an inherited tendency to store excessive body fat will manifest itself only when a sedentary lifestyle is combined with a high-fat diet. In this chapter we will examine the role of other dietary factors and see what effect they have on how much body fat is stored. First, however, you will need to grasp an important principle of nutrition science.

ADDITION EQUALS SUBTRACTION

One of the fundamental principles of nutrition science is that addition equals subtraction. Unfortunately, this principle is not widely appreciated even by many nutrition educators and registered dietitians. However, it is a principle that everyone who designs experimental diets must come to understand.

Since most dietitians do not conduct basic nutrition research and design experimental diets, it is understandable that many would never have encountered it. This has led to a lot of confusion about what happens when you subtract something from the diet. If what is being subtracted is a caloric ingredient, then this principle demands that an alternative caloric ingredient be added. Let's see how this principle applies to the L.A. Diet.

In Chapter 3 we saw why it was very important to replace fat calories with carbohydrate calories. In Chapter 6 you will learn why substituting protein for carbohydrate would not be wise. In Chapter 2 you learned how important it is to maintain body temperature. This means the energy provided by the fatty foods you eat must be replaced by other energy (caloric) sources, or you will become cold and hungry.

As we have seen, it is okay to lower the level of fuel in the fat storage tank only if you simultaneously increase the level of fuel in the carbohydrate (glycogen) storage tank. The addition of carbohydrates means the subtraction of fat. By eating more high-carbohydrate foods you will have less room for high-fat foods and will get more heat production out of fewer calories. This means you will need less insulation (subcutaneous fat stores).

CALORIC DENSITY

Caloric density refers to the concentration of calories in a food item. Since the calorie is a measure of heat energy, caloric density is sometimes referred to as *energy density*. In general, animal products and refined foods have a high caloric density or energy density, while plant foods have a low caloric density. Gorging foods have a high energy density, and grazing foods have a relatively low energy density.

The food items that have the highest caloric density are the refined fats and oils, with over 4,000 calories per pound, compared to pure sugar, which has about 1,700 calories per pound. Figure 5.1 shows how the amount of refined fats and oils has been increasing in the American

FIGURE 5.1

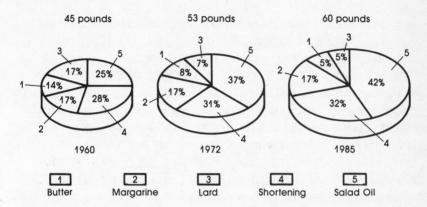

diet in the past 25 years. During this time the incidence of obesity has increased for nearly all age groups. Nothing will make you fatter than these refined fats and oils, because they are 100 percent fat calories.

Foods that provide a lot of bulk but few calories fill you up and leave little room in your stomach for foods with concentrated calories. For example, a pound of cheddar cheese has 1,805 calories, while a pound of carrots has 191 calories. You would have to eat nearly nine pounds of carrots to get the same number of calories you'd get from one pound of cheese. Since there is no way your stomach could hold nine pounds of anything, eating carrots instead of cheese would force you to eat meals with fewer calories more often.

Our reference man needs about 100 calories per hour to keep his metabolic furnace running. Assuming he sleeps 8 hours a night, he must consume all 2,400 calories in 16 waking hours, or 150 calories per hour. If he stuffed himself with 1½ pounds of cheese, he'd be set for the day. If he stuffed himself with 1½ pounds of carrots, he'd have to refuel again in just under 2 hours. Eating foods with a low caloric density all day long is what grazing is all about. Eating relatively small amounts of calorically or energy-dense foods two or three times a day is what gorging is all about.

Nibbling vs. Meal Eating

Years ago research showed that animals that ate a few large meals each day gained more weight than animals that ate the same amount of food by nibbling throughout the day. Eating large meals is known to elevate insulin levels. As we have already seen, insulin speeds up the burning of carbohydrates and shuts down the burning of fats. This means that meal eating promotes fat storage and carbohydrate burning. If you want to get rid of fat, it makes sense to eat a lot of small meals throughout the day. That is, in fact, what grazing—and the L.A. Diet Program—is all about.

I know that most psychologists and many dietitians still discourage eating between meals. Unfortunately, many dietitians, psychologists, and physicians involved in weight control who have not kept up with the latest scientific research or read this book may know less about getting rid of excess body fat and keeping it off than you now know. You may, however, still need their help in changing poor eating habits and overcoming temptations. If you have trouble going it alone, my advice is to give them this book and seek their guidance and support in switching from a gorging lifestyle to a grazing lifestyle.

Eating Slowly: A New Twist

One of the favorite behavioral tricks of psychologists who naively get involved in weight control is the admonition to eat slowly. How many overweight people have been told to put their fork down between bites? (Psychologists call this *time-energy displacement.*) Let's be realistic. How is this supposed to correct the metabolic imbalances created by a sedentary lifestyle and a high-fat diet? How are you going to carry on a normal conversation at mealtime if you have to count to 10 between bites?

Even if there is something to time-energy displacement, grazing is a much simpler and more rational way to limit the number of calories you consume over time. Why? Because eating low-caloric-density foods, like most vegetables and fruits, slows down the rate at which calories enter your body. If you switched from cheese to carrots, you would have to eat nine times faster to consume the same number of calories in, say, 15 minutes. Eating foods with a low caloric density achieves time-energy displacement without putting down your fork and counting to 10 between bites.

EFFECT OF CALORIC DENSITY
ON CALORIC INTAKE

A study conducted at the University of Alabama and published in *The American Journal of Clinical Nutrition* in May 1983 examined the effects of feeding the same subjects with diets differing in caloric density. Figure 5.2 shows the results.

Figure 5.2 shows the average caloric intake for subjects consuming either a high-energy-density diet (HED) or a low-energy-density diet (LED). Note that on the high-energy-density diet the subjects consumed an average of 3,000 calories per day. The same subjects consuming the low-energy-density diet (LED) averaged only 1,570 calories per day. It is important to note that the subjects in this study rated the two diets as being similar in producing satiety. They also rated the two diets as being equal in terms of palatability.

FIGURE 5.2

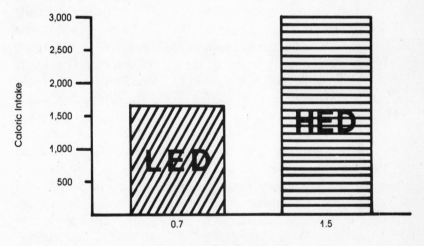

Calories per gram

This study demonstrated that what people eat is much more important than how they eat. On both diets subjects ate as much as they wanted of diets they found equally enjoyable. The only difference was that they ate 1,430 calories fewer each day on the low-caloric-density diet than the high-caloric-density diet. If it takes about 15 calories to keep each pound of body weight warm, this difference between the two diets would eventually translate into a weight loss of 95 pounds. How would you like to be able to lose that much excess baggage and not feel hungry all the time? That is the promise of the L.A. Diet.

It is important to note that this University of Alabama study lasted only five days, and it is possible that there could be some long-term adjustment to consuming a low-caloric-density diet. The low-caloric-density diet had a much higher crude fiber content (seven grams vs. one gram per 1,000 calories) as well as a different carbohydrate-to-fat ratio than the high-caloric-density diet. Research conducted by Dr. Lauren Lissner at Cornell University examined the effects of varying the caloric density only by reducing the percentage of calories from fat. Her results were in the *American Journal of Clinical Nutrition* in December 1987. She fed human subjects diets containing 15 to 20 percent, 30 to 35 percent, and 45 to 50 percent of their calories from fat. In Figure 5.3 we can see that on the highest-fat diet the subjects consumed nearly 700 calories per day more than on the low-fat diet. In Figure 5.4, from Dr. Lissner's study, we can see that there was no tendency to increase caloric intake with time on the low-fat (15 to 20 percent) diet, nor was there a trend to have decreasing caloric intake on the high-fat (45 to 50 percent) diet. It is not surprising, then, that on the high-fat diet the subjects were gaining weight, while on the low-fat diet they were losing weight. In the long run a 700-calorie per day deficit would translate into a weight difference of nearly 50 pounds.

Dr. Lissner's research is consistent with my observations of people's caloric intake while staying at the Pritikin Longevity Center in Santa Monica. The Pritikin diet, like the L.A. Diet, contains only about 10 percent fat. Skeptics have argued that people eat less on very low-fat diets because they are unpalatable. However, Dr. Lissner's research subjects rated the food items on the low-fat diet slightly more palatable than the high-fat diet. Dr. Lissner concluded "that habitual, unrestricted consumption of low-fat diets may be an effective approach to weight reduction." The L.A. Diet described in this book has about half the fat content of Dr. Lissner's low-fat diet and would predictably produce an even more dramatic drop in body fat.

FIGURE 5.3: ENERGY INTAKE

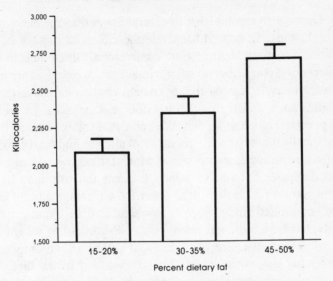

From **Am J Clin Nutr**, Dec. 1987, 886-892. Used with permission.

FIGURE 5.4: DAILY ENERGY INTAKE

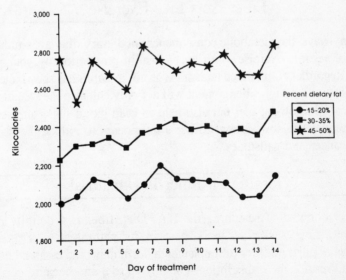

From **Am J Clin Nutr**, Dec. 1987, 886-892. Used with permission.

THE FIBER FACTOR

The L.A. Diet is also much higher in natural fibers than the diet used in Dr. Lissner's study. In order to separate the effects of dietary fat and dietary fiber, her study kept the fiber content of all three diets low.

The effects of dietary fiber on caloric intake and weight loss are much less dramatic than decreasing the fat content of the diet. Nevertheless, many studies have shown that dietary fiber can enhance the weight-reducing potential of a low-fat diet. We know that soluble dietary fibers can dramatically lower insulin production after a high-carbohydrate meal. Since insulin increases the rate at which the body burns carbohydrate and decreases the rate at which it burns fat, this may be the mechanism whereby high-fiber diets lower the set point for body fat. A recent well-controlled study suggests that soluble fiber found in fruits, beans, oats, barley, lentils, and many vegetables can aid in weight loss. Dr. Stevens at Cornell University found that caloric intake dropped by 153 calories per day when soluble fiber was added to the diet. This suggests that dietary fiber alone can reduce body fat stores by 10 to 15 pounds without any need to count calories or go hungry (*American Journal of Clinical Nutrition,* 1987; 46:812–7).

Fiber Acts Like Exercise

In many ways, the metabolic consequences of dietary fiber are similar to those of aerobic exercise. Both lower insulin production by your pancreas. Regardless of the mechanism involved, research has shown clearly that diets with a high fiber content will not only enhance the weight-loss potential of a low-fat diet but also help to keep blood sugar and serum cholesterol levels low. Dietary fiber also appears to reduce the risk of colon cancer and gallstones.

Gorging on Fiber Is Unnatural

When it comes to fine-tuning the L.A. Diet, fiber is a definite plus. However, fiber seems to work best in its natural state. Excessive amounts of purified fiber in supplemental form may bind essential nutrients and reduce their absorption. For this reason, and because concentrated fiber, like concentrated sugar or oils, is unnatural and fits our definition of gorging, we do not recommend fiber supplements. These supplements would be unnatural when separated from the whole grain or other source.

So, until we know more about the benefits and risks of fiber supplements, it seems wisest to simply eat natural foods high in fiber such as fruits, vegetables, grains, beans, and potatoes. Since these foods are also rich sources of other nutrients, there is little reason to be concerned about too much fiber creating deficiencies.

GORGING ON SALT

Since there are no calories in salt, most health professionals never warn people trying to lose weight to avoid salt. Recent research has shown that adding salt to a meal significantly increases insulin levels. As we have seen, anything that increases insulin levels tends to make you fat because insulin promotes fat storage and carbohydrate burning. Incidentally, high-fat diets tend to raise both insulin levels and blood pressure.

Salt is taboo on the L.A. Diet for many other reasons. For example, it is the primary cause of high blood pressure and strokes. You can easily get all the salt you need from natural foods, so there is no reason to supplement your diet with huge amounts of this nutrient.

WARMING UP TO HOT SPICES

One of the biggest surprises I had while searching the scientific literature for ways to fine-tune the L.A. Diet was the effects of "hot" spices. It never occurred to me that "whatever warms you up slims you down" would apply to spices as well as exercise. Nevertheless, a study conducted at Oxford Polytechnic in Oxford, England, proved just that. The researchers found a 25 percent greater increase in metabolic rate after a meal containing "hot" spices (chili and mustard) than after the same meal without the spices. Many people have noticed that hot spiced foods make them sweat and this may be why. In theory, this means that spicing up the L.A. Diet could enhance its weight reduction potential.

Since it is necessary to cut the salt out of your diet for both health and weight control reasons, we encourage you to experiment with spices in its place. Those who think grazing means dull eating are invited to try some of the "hot and spicy" recipes in Part III of this book.

GRAZING ON FERMENTED GRAINS AND GRAPES

The fermentation of grains and grapes gives us beer and wine. During fermentation much of the carbohydrate is converted to ethanol (alcohol). In the body, alcohol is metabolized as carbohydrate. It is not readily converted into fat. Alcohol has also been shown to raise the metabolic rate, which means greater heat production. Since the body can't store alcohol the way it does fat, it probably does not make you fat. However, having as little as one or two drinks a day has been shown to double your risk of having a stroke.

Alcohol also increases your chances of cirrhosis of the liver and certain types of cancer. In addition, alcohol has a very high caloric density. Each gram of alcohol has seven calories, compared to four calories per gram for sugar. Given the high caloric density of alcohol, it seems an unwise choice for a weight-control plan.

In addition to those health concerns, alcohol also creates psychological problems because it is a drug. While the L.A. Diet keeps you from being driven to overeat, it does not keep you from being tempted. You don't need me to tell you that alcohol makes it much more difficult to resist temptation. If alcohol is used, it should never be on an empty stomach while waiting to be seated at a restaurant.

HOW TO SWEETEN THE GRAZING DIET

At first glance, pure white sugar crystals would appear to be a safe addition to the L.A. Diet. After all, there is no fat in sugar. However, there also are no vitamins or minerals or fiber. It is the worst of "empty calorie" foods. Also, a pound of sugar has over 1,700 calories. A pound of bananas has only 400–450 calories by comparison.

Sugar is also "unnatural" in the sense that we were not designed by nature to be exposed to such an intense hedonic stimulus. Monkeys and gorillas also love sugar, but they never find any in the jungle. Given its high caloric density and unnatural pleasure intensity, it is not surprising that experimental animals tend to stuff themselves with sugar when they are sitting around bored all day in a little cage. And eating for stimulation may overcome the body's natural feedback mechanism, that normally prevents the overconsumption of a low-fat diet. When sugar is converted into fat, about 25% of the heat is lost. This would normally raise the metabolic rate enough to shut down the appetite by warming you up. However, in the study of caged animals, the availability of refined sugar or the addition of sugar to the normal diet results in the excessive consumption of calories and obesity. This occurs even though the animals' metabolic rate is chronically elevated.

For people who are very active, there is probably little danger in including a modest amount of refined sugar in the diet, even though it is not recommended. However, if you are sedentary and often bored, it is likely that the addition of sugar to the L.A. Diet will undermine your success.

Another problem with sugar and other refined carbohydrates is that they lack fiber, which means they will elevate insulin levels more than naturally occurring carbohydrate.

If you have a high set point for body fat, it would be best to restrict your sweet tooth to fresh and frozen fruit. The use of even fruit juices and fruit juice concentrates should be kept to a minimum because most of the fiber has been removed. If you are at or below your "ideal" body weight, the use of fruit juice concentrates as sweeteners would be acceptable.

Artificial Sweeteners

Artificial sweeteners have been proven to be of no use in aiding weight loss. In fact, some researchers have found small but significant weight gains in people using them. Why this has occurred is not clear. They may operate like sugar and trigger overeating because they trigger an innate pleasure center that causes us to continue eating for the sake of pleasurable stimulation.

Some research also suggests they can trigger the reflex release of insulin. Just as the smell of food triggers your salivary juices to flow, a sweet taste may trigger your pancreas to release insulin. Our bodies were not designed to handle false hedonic stimuli. In the past a sweet taste was always accompanied by sugar, so it made sense for the body to prepare for this incoming fuel by increasing the insulin level. In an artificial situation our natural reactions would be inappropriate.

Addictive drugs, such as cocaine and heroin, certainly set up a false hedonic response because they trigger an innate pleasure center. Most people who drink alcohol or use cocaine do not become addicted, so it is likely that most people can use artificial sweeteners or refined sugars in small amounts occasionally with little or no danger. However, if you are one of those people who reacts to sweeetness as an alcoholic reacts to alcohol, it would be best for you to abstain completely from using anything with a concentrated sweet taste except whole fruit.

VITAMINS AND MINERALS

Nutritional deficiencies do not occur when a variety of natural foods are eaten in amounts that meet your energy needs. On the L.A. Diet you are in little danger of developing any nutritional deficiency.

Too Much of a Good Thing Is Bad

The food supplement industry has been fairly successful in conning people into believing that if a little is good, more must be better. They have gotten a lot of people to believe that if a little is needed to make you healthy, then more will make you superhealthy. There is simply no scientific support for these notions.

Can Supplements Undo the Harm Caused by Gorging?

The real danger of the claims made for supplements is that people like the myth that supplements are a form of "health insurance" for people who don't always eat right. Most people who gorge and are sedentary would much prefer to take a magic pill that would "melt off the pounds" or "clean out their arteries" without changing their ways. To be honest, I would quickly abandon the L.A. Diet Program if such a supplement really existed. Unfortunately, it doesn't.

People who gorge and take large amounts of vitamins and minerals are simply adding insult to injury. Indeed, megadosing on vitamin and mineral supplements is a form of gorging. The scientific evidence clearly shows that Americans are dying from dietary excesses, not deficiencies. What sense does it make to add excesses of vitamins and minerals to other dietary excesses?

HOW TO CHEAT AND SURVIVE

Any deviation from the L.A. Diet entails some health risks for most people. Nevertheless, this risk is not spread evenly throughout the population. The amount of risk you incur by deviating from the L.A. Diet depends on inherited predispositions to develop various degenerative diseases. Only a thorough physical examination coupled with appropriate medical tests and an assessment of your medical history and that of your family can help you to play the odds in your favor.

Each of us is born with genetic strengths and weaknesses. Some of us tend to gain body fat much more easily than others. If you gain weight easily, it is very important for you to avoid all calorically dense foods, especially those with a high fat content. If high blood pressure runs in your family, it is relatively more important for you to avoid high-salt foods. If your serum cholesterol is well above average, it is more important for you to avoid foods high in saturated fats and cholesterol such as eggs, cheese, and red meats than it is for you to avoid almonds and olive oil (unless you're also overfat).

If you gain weight easily, you may be better off with turkey than a fatty fish like mackerel or salmon. However, if you are naturally thin but have a tendency to form blood clots, salmon would probably be a wiser choice than turkey, because fish oils reduce the tendency for blood to clot.

Someone with a high serum cholesterol level whose father and older brother had heart attacks in their forties would be ill-advised to exceeed the L.A. Diet's recommendation for animal products such as meats, eggs, cheese, butter, and ice cream. Someone with no family history of heart disease and a low serum cholesterol could exceed the L.A. Diet's limits on shrimp and eggs from time to time with much less risk of developing clogged arteries. (Notice that I said "much less risk" and not "no risk." As far as we know, foods high in saturated fats and/or cholesterol increase everyone's risk of developing atherosclerosis [clogged arteries]. But research has shown that certain risk factors make it far more dangerous for some people to gorge on foods rich in saturated fats and cholesterol than for others.)

Risk Factor Assessment
Is the Key to Low-Risk Cheating

Another example of how you can play the odds in your favor would be a 60-year-old woman with low blood pressure and no family history of high blood pressure. She would be taking a much smaller chance exceeding the L.A. Diet guidelines for sodium than a young woman whose parents both have high blood pressure. This doesn't mean there is no risk, because excess salt may also increase the risk of developing stomach cancer and osteoporosis quite independently of causing high blood pressure. Nevertheless, the main danger of too much sodium is high blood pressure.

If you are very lean even while gorging, you may be able to eat a bit more high-fat vegetable foods such as avocados, nuts, and seeds with relatively few health risks compared to someone who stores body fat efficiently. On the other hand, if you're lean but have a strong family history of high blood pressure, you may be taking a bigger chance gorging on salty foods than on almonds and avocados. A man who inherits a tendency to store fat easily may be blessed with kidneys that get rid of excess salt so efficiently that he could get away with gorging on salt but not on nuts and avocados.

The point to be made here is that it is best for most people to stick close to the L.A. Diet guidelines. They represent my best guess of what will produce optimal health for most people. It is based on an extensive review of the scientific literature, as well as my own research and clinical experience. It is not just another fad diet that must be followed religiously in order to gain eternal youth. Cheating or simply deviating from these guidelines occasionally will not cause you to drop dead tomorrow.

Minor digressions from the L.A. Diet are relatively meaningless in the long run for most people. And remember, you *will* be tempted occasionally. When you are, keep in mind that these urges are simply temptations, which you can handle, and not drives, which no one can resist. Other weight control plans leave you *biologically driven* to eat; the L.A. Diet can't prevent you from being tempted, but it won't leave you with a real biological *need* to deviate from its guidelines.

Stress Does Not Cause Overeating

One thing to keep in mind, especially when you are just starting on the L.A. Diet and may fear "failure," is that stress does not cause overeating. Many dieters have become convinced that stressful events cause them to overeat or blow their diet, and in a sense stress does trigger a binge. But in reality, very few people actually overeat because of stress. Stress simply undermines the intellect or will of people who are chronically undereating a high-fat diet. Once their intellect is focused on another, more threatening problem, their biological need for more fuel is freed from its intellectual constraints. When this happens, they binge or chronically overeat until they have regained all their lost weight. They return to their normal set point for body fat.

Your Health Is Your Responsibility

It is, of course, your life, and you have a right to live it as you see fit. In order to make rational decisions about any aspect of your life you must be knowledgeable about their probable long-term effects. This is especially true when it comes to your health. You can do much more to assure yourself a long and healthy life than the best doctors can. Why people get sick and die is becoming less mysterious and more preventable all the time. But prevention requires application of this scientific evidence to your lifestyle.

Except for getting rid of excess body fat, the advice in this book is, by necessity, somewhat general. It is not meant to replace the individual guidance of caring and knowledgeable health professionals. You will need their expertise in risk factor assessment and their clinical judgment in order to best assess the extent of the risk you will be taking by ignoring the L.A. Diet's guidelines for a healthy diet and lifestyle. If you want to cheat and survive, have your physician evaluate your health status to make sure you are keeping your risk factors within acceptable limits. An ounce of prevention is truly worth a pound of cure when it comes to heart disease, strokes, and cancer.

6
PUTTING THE PROTEIN MYTH
OUT TO PASTURE

Americans have had a long love affair with protein. Their admiration for protein stems from unsubstantiated claims promoted primarily by the dairy, egg, and meat industries. We have been warned about the dangers of not getting enough protein and told that beef gives strength. It does not. We have been told that only milk, eggs, and meats have "complete" proteins and that vegetable proteins are "incomplete" and must be carefully combined in order to get adequate amounts of all the essential amino acids (the building blocks of proteins).

In the 1960s and '70s, high-protein, low-carbohydrate diets, modified fasting supplemented by liquid and powdered protein, and similar diets became the rage for quick weight loss. You may recall the Atkins Diet, the Stillman Diet, the Drinking Man's Diet, the Mayo Clinic Diet, the Grapefruit Diet, and the Calories Don't Count Diet, to name but a few. They are all examples of low-carbohydrate, high-protein diets. It was during these "protein years," from about 1950 to the mid-1970s, that deaths from heart disease peaked in this country.

SCIENTIFIC SUPPORT FOR THE "WONDERS" OF PROTEIN WAS LACKING

The scientific support for our love affair with protein was underwhelming at best. As we shall see, Americans have been conned into believing they need lots of animal protein to stay strong and healthy. The great protein myth was the basis for convincing most Americans that gorging is the basis for a "balanced" diet. In reality, our paranoia about getting enough high-quality protein led to an epidemic of heart disease and many other nutritional disasters including obesity.

In order to understand where protein fits into the L.A. Diet you will need to know a few things about what protein is and how it is metabolized and utilized by the body. In the process we will dispel a few of the more prevalent myths about the need for dietary protein.

AMINO ACIDS ARE THE BUILDING BLOCKS OF PROTEINS

The human body is about 15 to 20 percent protein by weight. Proteins come in many shapes and sizes, but they are all composed of the same 22 building blocks known as *amino acids.* Just as the body strings together several hundred sugar (glucose) molecules to make glycogen (animal starch), the body also strings together amino acids to make proteins. But proteins are not simply stored energy.

Proteins, unlike glycogen and triglyceride, do not serve the body primarily as a source of stored energy between meals even though they can be used in this way in an emergency. All proteins, even though made up of the same amino acids, differ tremendously in their physical and chemical properties, depending on the sequence and ratio of the amino acids they contain. Some proteins, such as hair (keratin) and collagen (found in ligaments and tendons), are structural. All enzymes are proteins, and many hormones, such as insulin, are proteins. Actin and myosin are the two contractile proteins in muscles that move us about.

In short, proteins are the machinery of life. This is their primary function in the body. In order to synthesize these proteins, your body needs 22 amino acids. Our bodies can make most of these amino acids, so it is not essential that they be present in the diet. This is why they are termed *nonessential* amino acids. However, there are nine amino acids that cannot be synthesized in the body and must, therefore, be supplied in the diet. These are called the *essential* amino acids.

In general, the proteins found in animals are similar in their amino acid content to those produced by the human body. Plant proteins, by contrast, are more likely to differ considerably in amino acid content from those produced in the human body. This is not surprising when you consider that animal proteins serve functions similar to those in our bodies, while the proteins in plants perform much different functions. Because of this the protein content of animal foods has a better ratio of these essential amino acids than the proteins found in plants. In order to dramatize this difference, animal proteins were called "complete" and vegetable proteins "incomplete."

"COMPLETE" AND "INCOMPLETE" PROTEIN: THE PROTEIN HOAX

In order to get enough "complete" protein the average American gorges on about 190 pounds of red meat, 65 pounds of poultry, 15 pounds of fish, 250 eggs, 20 pounds of cheese, and 260 pounds of other dairy products each year. Yet we actually don't need those gorging foods in our quest for "complete" protein. One of the leading authorities on amino acid and protein requirements is Dr. Alfred Harper, chairman of the Nutritional Sciences Department at the University of Wisconsin and past chairman of the Food and Nutrition Board of the National Research Council. According to Dr. Harper,

> One of the biggest fallacies ever perpetrated is that there is any need for so-called complete protein. Some proteins provide more limited amounts of some amino acids than others. But it has been recognized since the start of this century that if you increase the quantity, you don't have to worry about quality. We have shown that adults can remain in protein balance on a diet of wheat, even [white] flour.

Table 6.1 lists the amounts of each of the essential amino acids found in a variety of animal and vegetable foods. You can see that pasta made from white flour contains all of the essential amino acids. In fact, the proteins of both animals and vegetables contain all of the essential amino acids. There is no such thing as a naturally occurring vegetable protein that does not contain *all* of the essential amino acids.

TABLE 6.1. The Essential Amino Acid Content of Selected Plant and Animal Foods Compared to That Required by an Adult Man

Essential Amino Acids	Amount Required mg/day	Amount Contained in 500 Cal. of:					
		Milk mg	Beef mg	Corn mg	Bean mg	Pasta mg	Spinach mg
Phe + Tyr	1,000	2,485	3,102	1,279	2,974	1,484	3,440
Isoleucine	700	1,592	2,162	555	1,801	873	2,140
Leucine	1,000	2,456	3,383	1,556	2,724	1,155	3,520
Valine	700	1,713	2,296	613	1,923	990	2,520
Met + Cys	800	835	1,547	378	634	593	1,700
Threonine	500	1,150	1,824	479	1,373	679	2,040
Tryptophan	250	350	482	73	295	204	740
Lysine	800	1,942	3,611	346	2,352	562	2,840

Based on *FAO Nutrition Meetings Report* Series, No. 522, Rome, 1973.

Quality and Quantity Confusion

You can see from Table 6.1 that just 500 calories of milk and beef will supply more than enough of all the essential amino acids. You will note that the ratio of the essential amino acids in these foods is close to the ratio of essential amino acids required by an adult man (requirements for women are even lower). This is why they are referred to as "high-quality" proteins. You may also be surprised to learn that 500 calories of spinach supplies a greater amount of all the essential amino acids (except lysine and isoleucine) than the same amount of calories from milk or beef. The reason for this is shown in Table 6.2.

In Table 6.2 you can see why spinach is so high in all of the essential amino acids. It contains 40 percent of its calories as protein, whereas corn, for example, has only 10 percent protein calories. But comparing

TABLE 6.2. THE PERCENTAGE OF CALORIES FROM PROTEIN, FAT, AND
CARBOHYDRATE IN SELECTED FOODS

Food Items	PRO % Cal	FAT % Cal	CHO % Cal	PRO (g) per 500 Cal
Milk (whole)	21	48	31	27
Beef (ground chuck)	35	65	0	43
Corn (grits)	10	3	87	12
Bean (red kidney)	24	4	72	32
Pasta (Durem wheat)	14	3	83	17
Spinach (raw)	40	10	50	50

50 grams of protein from spinach with 12 grams of protein from corn is obviously not a fair comparison. If our reference man were to consume 50 grams of corn protein, he would get an adequate amount of all the essential amino acids.

Protein quality comes into play only when the quantity of protein in the diet is very low. For example, you can see in Table 6.1 that 500 calories of milk (about three cups) would supply all of the essential amino acids an average man needs. However, 500 calories from beans would fall short on the sulfur amino acids (Met + Cys).

In Table 6.2 you can see that this is a more than fair comparison since we are comparing the amounts of essential amino acids in only 27 grams of milk protein with 32 grams of bean protein. In other words, 27 grams of high-quality milk protein supplies all of the essential amino acids a man needs, but even 32 grams of bean protein supplies only 80 percent of the required amount of sulfur amino acids.

Of course, no one eats just 500 calories a day for long. It would take just over 40 grams of bean protein to supply a man with all the essential amino acids he needs. This means only 650 calories of beans would supply all the essential amino acids in adequate amounts. Since an average man consumes over 2,000 calories per day, we can see that even corn would supply an adequate amount of all the essential amino acids. Why? We would have to multiply the amounts of amino acids from corn in Table 6.1 by four-plus if our reference man ate nothing but corn.

The Most Limiting Amino Acid
Determines Need for Protein Quantity

The most limiting amino acid in corn is tryptophan. The 73 milligrams supplied by 500 calories of corn is far short of the 250 milligrams needed by an adult man. Nevertheless, if 2,000 calories of corn were eaten, that would supply 292 milligrams of tryptophan ($4 \times 73 = 292$), which is more than the 250 milligrams required.

From this discussion it should be clear that it is all but impossible to fail to meet your needs for all of the essential amino acids by eating only a single source of "incomplete" vegetable protein. I know this sounds like heresy to those who were taught that only by carefully combining different vegetable protein sources could they satisfy their protein needs. The facts prove otherwise.

How did all that high-quality protein get into the meat, milk, and eggs in the first place? Cows and chickens don't eat meat. All of the essential amino acids in eggs were originally present in the grains consumed by the chicken, and yet eggs are considered the "highest-quality" protein there is. Gorillas and elephants can get all the protein they need by grazing, so why should we think we need meat, eggs, and milk to get big and strong?

PROTEIN MAKES YOU FAT

Table 6.2 also shows the percentage of calories from fats and carbohydrates. Note that the animal products (beef and milk) are loaded with fat while the vegetable foods contain most of their calories as carbohydrate. In fact, most high-protein foods are high in fat (e.g., nuts, eggs, meats, cheese, milk, soybeans, seeds, and some, but not all, fish). These are gorging foods. From the grazing viewpoint they are the most fattening foods you can eat except the refined fats and oils like butter, margerine, vegetable oils, shortening, lard, chocolate, and cream.

Fish, poultry, egg whites, and nonfat dairy products are the preferred sources of animal protein on the L.A. Diet because they are relatively low in fat. Nevertheless, they must be eaten in moderation because too much protein, like too much fat, can promote obesity.

The scientific research that demonstrates that fat makes you fat is overwhelming. However, there is also some evidence linking high-protein diets with the deposition of excess body fat. Table 6.3 shows the final body weight and fat content of rats fed a low- (5 percent) and high- (25 percent) protein diet. In both cases the rats ate as much as they wanted. The rats eating the high-protein diet were bigger and 50 percent fatter than the rats consuming the low-protein diet.

TABLE 6.3. FINAL BODY WEIGHT AND BODY FAT OF RATS FED AD LIBITUM LOW- AND HIGH-PROTEIN DIETS OF EQUAL CALORIC CONTENT

Protein in Diet (%)	Body Weight (g)	Body Fat (%)
5	397	16
25	487	24

Science, 1981 (211:185–6)

Fat-Forming Amino Acids

In experimental animals, increasing dietary protein increases body fat. The reason for this is not clear. However, we do know that the amino acids are metabolized via two biochemical pathways. Most are metabolized as if they were carbohydrates (glucogenic or glucose-forming), but many of the essential amino acids (lysine, isoleucine, leucine, phenylalanine, and tyrosine) are metabolized like fat (ketogenic or fat-forming).

Excessive Protein Makes You Fat

Your body does not store extra protein as it does extra fat or carbohydrate. This means that any excess of these ketogenic amino acids can easily increase the body's fat stores. Since the ketogenic amino acids represent about 35 percent of the total, a high-protein diet would be very close to the typical American diet, with about 40 percent of its calories from fat. In 1967, Dr. Miller published a study showing that human subjects gained weight more easily from excess protein than from excess carbohydrates (*American Journal of Clinical Nutrition,* 1967; 20:1212–22). While this research is far from conclusive, it does indicate a mechanism whereby high-protein diets can make you fat.

7

HOW THE L.A. DIET PROGRAM CAN KEEP YOU HEALTHY FOR LIFE

The dangers of gorging are not limited to making you fat. If this were the case, the L.A. Diet would simply be a great way to lose excess body fat and keep it off. It is much more than that. As you will see in this chapter, gorging can kill you even if it doesn't make you fat. Grazing, on the other hand, is an excellent approach to diet that can promote good health for your entire family, regardless of their weight.

Even naturally thin individuals or those who stay thin by doing heavy work and/or lots of exercise can benefit from adopting the L.A. Diet. Gorging is the primary cause of deaths from heart attacks, diabetes, high blood pressure, strokes, and most of the more common types of cancer. It is also a causal factor in a host of other less deadly health problems from hemorrhoids and constipation to tooth decay and hearing loss. By switching to a grazing lifestyle you will maximize your chances of leading a long and healthy life.

GOVERNMENT GUIDELINES
FOR A HEALTHY DIET

In recent years the National Academy of Science's NRC Committee on Diet, Nutrition, and Cancer issued its dietary guidelines for reducing the risk of cancer. These guidelines were very similar to those issued jointly by the U.S. Department of Health and Human Services and the U.S. Department of Agriculture. The American Heart Association, the American Cancer Society, and the National Cancer Institute have also made similar recommendations after reviewing the scientific literature. All of these guidelines encourage Americans to modify their diets in order to reduce their risk of developing cancer, heart disease, stroke, and other serious illnesses. The L.A. Diet meets or exceeds all of the recommendations made by these organizations. Let's take a brief look at the recommendations and how the L.A. Diet follows them.

1. EAT A VARIETY OF FOODS.

No single food contains all of the nutrients you need. By eating a variety of foods from the different food groups you will be reasonably assured of getting an adequate supply of all essential nutrients; you will also reduce your chances of being exposed to a significant amount of naturally occurring toxins and carcinogens (cancer-causing substances) in any one food. The L.A. Diet offers you a choice of many low-fat foods, such as fruits, vegetables, grains, beans, nonfat dairy products, and lean meats, poultry, and fish.

2. AVOID TOO MUCH FAT, SATURATED FAT, AND CHOLESTEROL.

Excess dietary fat has been associated with the development of most of the more common forms of cancer and heart disease. Gorging on foods high in saturated fat and/or cholesterol is the primary cause of clogged arteries, which account for half of all deaths in the United States. When you switch to grazing, on the average, your serum cholesterol should drop about 25 to 30 percent within a month.

If you follow the L.A. Diet starting early in life, your chances of ever dying from clogged arteries will be close to zero. Only those rare individuals who inherit a serious metabolic defect in handling blood lipids will be in danger. Grazing promises to virtually eliminate this country's number-one killer without drugs, surgery, or miracles.

The L.A. Diet encourages the generous consumption of fruits and vegetables. Numerous lines of scientific inquiry lead to the conclusion that increasing the amounts of fruits and vegetables in the diet will help to lower serum cholesterol due to their high pectin content. In addition, fruits and vegetables are rich sources of carotene, vitamins, fibers, and other compounds that prevent or reduce the development of cancers in experimental animals. Research also shows that people who consume more fruits and vegetables have a much lower risk of developing many types of cancer.

3. EAT FOODS WITH ADEQUATE STARCH AND FIBER.
4. AVOID TOO MUCH SUGAR.

These two guidelines are combined because they are really the same guideline. In grazing terminology the admonition is to eat unrefined carbohydrate foods in place of refined carbohydrates. This means fruit instead of sugar and whole grain breads, cereals, and pasta instead of white rice, white bread, and white pasta. In other words, eat foods closer to the way they come from nature than after the food processors get through with them. Refining leads to unnatural foods. Gorging includes the consumption of foods stripped of their natural fibers and other nutrients.

Increased dietary fiber probably helps prevent cancer of the colon, lowers serum cholesterol levels, and improves blood sugar regulation, which means that the L.A. Diet is ideal for most diabetics. However, the L.A. Diet will require a significant decrease in the drugs used to control a diabetic's blood sugar level. For this reason, diabetics should consult their physician and/or registered dietitian about how to go from gorging to grazing.

5. AVOID TOO MUCH SALT.

Salt is undoubtedly the primary cause of high blood pressure. Last year the American Heart Association recommended that we all restrict our sodium intake to 1,000 milligrams per 1,000 calories. This is the same guideline used in the recipes in this book. The only difference between the L.A. Diet and AHA guidelines for sodium is the upper limit. The AHA allows up to 3 grams of sodium daily, while the L.A. Diet limits sodium intake to 1.5 grams per day. This lower limit is certainly safer for salt-sensitive people and those who already have high blood pressure. There is no known danger from limiting sodium to 500 to 1,500 milligrams per day.

Our preference for salty foods is learned, and research has shown that people lose their taste for salt in a few months if they avoid it religiously. When you first stop using salt, food will seem bland and tasteless. After you have avoided salt for several months, the same foods will begin to taste much better. Most people who successfully kick the salt habit report that food tastes much better to them without salt than it used to with salt before they quit. This is not surprising since it is our taste for salt that is unnatural.

6. IF YOU DRINK ALCOHOL, DO SO IN MODERATION

Alcohol is the major cause of cirrhosis of the liver. It also causes birth defects and is best avoided entirely by pregnant women. Heavy drinking can also contribute to strokes and high blood pressure, and cancer of the throat and neck are much more common in heavy drinkers (especially if they also smoke).

Alcoholic beverages are poor sources of vitamins and minerals. Distilled spirits are essentially nutrient-free and should be consumed rarely, if at all. While several glasses of wine or beer per week pose little danger, the L.A. Diet does not encourage drinking alcoholic beverages.

By following these guidelines, you can maintain a healthy diet. And with the L.A. Diet, you can have enjoyable meals and better health for life.

8
GETTING STARTED: WHAT TO EXPECT

For most people the switch form a high-fat, low-fiber diet to the L.A. Diet will result in a wide array of biochemical and physiological changes. So far I've discussed why these changes occur. In this chapter I would like to tell you how these changes will affect your body—in short, what you will experience.

One of the most dramatic and easily observed changes will be a gradual loss of body fat. However, how quickly you lose body fat and how this fat loss translates into weight loss on the scale can be a bit tricky, especially during the first week or two. Many people become discouraged if they do not see a sudden and dramatic drop in body weight during the first week. These people may have experienced rapid weight loss in the past but did not realize that a large percentage of the weight they were losing was water, glycogen, and/or lean (not fatty) tissue. Unfortunately, this type of rapid weight loss is almost always short-lived and is never good for your health in the long run.

HOW MANY POUNDS OF FAT WILL
YOU LOSE PER WEEK?

You will recall that a pound of body fat represents about 3,500 calories of stored heat energy. As we have seen from the work of Dr. Lissner at Cornell University, simply cutting the percentage of calories from fat will automatically reduce caloric intake by 500 to 1,000 calories per day, which will result in the loss of one to two pounds of body fat per week. Increasing dietary fiber and reducing the caloric density of your meals by eating lots of soups and salads will also produce a consistent drop in appetite and, therefore, caloric intake.

In addition to the weight loss produced by the diet, regular aerobic exercise will also burn up stored body fat. How much fat is burned up during exercise will vary from person to person. For example, a 175-pound person who walks five miles per day for one week, will burn up about 3,500 calories or the equivalent of energy stored in one pound of body fat. Of course some of these calories will be from stored carbohydrate (glycogen). Loss of glycogen will increase your appetite somewhat, so the expected weight loss from this much exercise would be less than one pound per week.

Weight loss will also depend on body size. If two people, one weighing 350 pounds and another weighing 175 pounds, walk the same number of miles per day, and both make the same dietary changes, the 350-pound person will lose body fat at a rate at least twice that of the smaller person because it takes twice as much heat energy to keep a 350-pound person warm as it does to keep a 175-pound person warm. It also takes twice as much mechanical energy to move a 350-pound body one mile as it does a 175-pound body.

Depending on body size and how much exercise you do, you can expect to lose anywhere from one to perhaps four or five pounds of body fat per week with the L.A. Diet. That's not bad when you consider that this will happen without counting calories or going hungry. Of course fat loss does not always equal weight loss in the short run. When weight loss is faster than fat loss, people sometimes develop an excessively optimistic attitude about future losses, only to become discouraged later when weight loss slows down. Conversely, people whose weight loss is less than their fat loss in the beginning may become very discouraged. In this case they may abandon the diet simply because the scale is misleading them. It is very important to stick to the diet and exercise program *regardless* of what the scale says.

HOW THE SCALE CAN LIE ABOUT YOUR FAT LOSS

There are several reasons why fat loss does not equal weight loss, particularly during the first few weeks:

1. Switching to a high-carbohydrate diet will cause your muscles and liver to store more glycogen. (Remember that glycogen is a starchy substance that attracts water.) Athletes may gain five to six pounds of weight by carbohydrate-loading before a marathon. While it is unlikely that your glycogen stores will increase by more than 500 to 1,000 calories, this increase would still equal a weight gain of one or two pounds. This means you can lose two pounds of fat and gain two pounds of stored glycogen during the first week, and the scale will tell you nothing happened. After the first week your glycogen stores will plateau, so they will not keep you from losing weight.

2. Women during their reproductive years will experience a weight gain of two to five pounds during the second half of their menstrual cycle. This gain is primarily fluid. Nevertheless, if you start this program in mid-cycle, the bathroom scale will tell you nothing happened in the first two weeks even though you lost five pounds of body fat.

3. Regular aerobic exercise will expand your circulatory system's capacity. This means more and bigger blood vessels and an increase in blood volume of up to 30 percent. Since about 5 to 6 percent of the body weight is blood, we would expect a weight gain of two to five pounds, depending on body size. This usually occurs gradually during the first month or two as your body adapts to regular aerobic exercise. On the scale this could wipe out as much as a pound of body fat loss per week during the first month. In addition, exercise may also increase muscle mass. This is particularly true for men who add calisthenics or weight training to their exercise regimen.

4. The high fiber content of the L.A. Diet will increase the amount of fluid held in your gut. Even on a standard American diet people typi-

cally gain from one to four pounds during the day. On the L.A. Diet you may experience an additional weight gain of one to two pounds during the later part of the day. You may also experience a little more bloating in your stomach and lower abdomen from the extra dietary fiber. Your body will adjust to this after a while. In the meantime it is very important for you to realize you are not getting a potbelly. It will be gone in the morning.

Your digestive tract is designed to handle this extra fiber. High fiber not only helps you lose weight in the long run but also reduces problems like constipation and hemorrhoids. The likelihood of more serious health problems like colon cancer and diverticulosis is also greatly diminished by the extra dietary fiber you will be consuming on the L.A. Diet.

There are also several factors that may cause your scale to tell you you are losing more weight than your actual fat loss represents:

1. The L.A. Diet is low in salt. In some people salt causes the retention of fluid. When you switch from a high-salt to a low-salt diet, you may experience a fluid loss of one to three pounds. This loss of fluid will occur during the first few days. Nevertheless, it may result in a much greater weight loss than fat loss during the first week. This can leave you with unrealistic expectations for future weight loss, which can lead to disappointment because it seems that the diet isn't working as well as it did during the first week.

2. If you are working up a good sweat while exercising, you may temporarily dehydrate yourself. Since each pint of sweat weighs a pound, losing a quart or two exercising on a hot day can cause a fluid loss of two to four pounds. This water loss can sometimes accumulate over a period of several days, particularly in older people, whose thirst mechanism is sometimes blunted. Since dehydration is unhealthy, it is a good idea to weigh yourself before and after exercising. For each pound you lose, drink a pint of water to restore your fluid balance. Remember, you would have to run 35 miles to burn up a pound of body fat, which means almost all the weight you lose exercising on a warm day is water that should be replaced.

The net effect of all these factors will vary considerably from one person to the next. It is certainly possible to lose five or six pounds of body fat in the first two weeks on this program and have the bathroom scale tell you your weight is the same. Conversely, you may lose only one pound of body fat the first week, but the scale will tell you you've lost five pounds. This is why it is so important not to get discouraged or overly optimistic about the rate at which you'll lose excess body fat on this program.

In general, younger people lose faster than older people. Men lose faster than women, and taller and fatter people lose faster than shorter people with less body fat. Obviously, people who exercise longer and more frequently also tend to lose weight more quickly. A 6'5" 28-year-old man weighing 350 pounds who does one or two hours of exercise a day could easily average four to five pounds of fat loss per week on this program. By contrast, a 5' 55-year-old woman weighing 130 pounds who can manage only 30 minutes of light exercise three or four times per week would lose closer to one pound of body fat per week.

WEIGHT LOSS WILL SLOW AS YOU APPROACH YOUR NEW SET POINT

After the first month or so, your weight loss will tend to stabilize and become more predictable. Eventually, depending on how much extra body fat you initially had, you will begin to reach a new set point for your body weight. As this occurs, your weekly weight loss will diminish gradually until it plateaus at the weight of the new you. As long as you continue to graze and exercise, your body fat will not come back, and you will never have to count calories or go hungry again. Of course, you must remember that you are what you eat. If you start eating more dietary fat, it will most assuredly accumulate on your hips, thighs, and stomach—just as it did before.

OTHER CHANGES TO EXPECT

In addition to causing a dramatic drop in body fat, the L.A. Diet Program will have a variety of other physiological and biochemical effects. Since the L.A. Diet is a nutritionally balanced diet, you do not have to check with your doctor before starting this program, provided you are in reasonably good health. However, if you are under a doctor's care, it would be wise to inform your physician about your decision to switch from an unhealthy gorging diet to the L.A. Diet. This is particularly true if you have any of the following conditions.

DIABETES

The American Diabetes Association now recommends a low-fat, high-fiber diet for diabetics. Research by Dr. James Anderson at the University of Kentucky and at the Pritikin Longevity Center in Santa Monica has shown that most Type II diabetics can be controlled without medication on a low-fat, high-fiber diet. This means that diabetics taking insulin or oral hypoglycemic agents should tell their doctors that they will have to have their medication reduced when they start this program. Eventually most will be able to control their blood sugar without insulin or oral agents, but *this should be done only under medical supervision.*

HYPERLIPIDEMIA

The high-fat American diet causes an excessive buildup of cholesterol and/or triglycerides (lipids) in the blood. Last October the National Heart, Lung and Blood Institute launched the National Cholesterol Education Program. This program is currently trying to educate physicians and the general public about the dangers of elevated blood lipids (hyperlipidemia). A serum cholesterol above 200 milligrams per deciliter is now clearly associated with increased risk of heart attacks. Many health professionals believe an ideal blood cholesterol level is under 160 milligrams per deciliter.

Research at the Pritikin Longevity Center and in Denmark (*American Journal of Clinical Nutrition,* August 1986; 44:212–9) has clearly shown that the vast majority of people with undesirably high blood lipids can lower them to a safe level by adopting a low-fat, low-cholesterol, high-fiber diet. Most people currently taking drugs to control their hyperlipidemia could have their blood lipids adequately controlled simply by adopting the L.A. Diet. People taking drugs to control dangerously high blood lipids should talk to their doctors about the possibility of controlling their hyperlipidemia with the L.A. Diet. The Danish study conducted by Dr. Lief Thuesen at the University Department of Cardiology, Aarhus Hospital, found a 41 percent drop in LDL-cholesterol (the "bad" cholesterol) on a diet similar to the L.A. Diet.

This drop is as good or better than that observed with the most potent cholesterol lowering drugs but without the dangers of adverse side effects you can get with drugs.

HYPERTENSION

High blood pressure is primarily the result of consuming the high-salt, high-fat American diet. Before there were drugs to control high blood pressure, Dr. Kempner at Duke University used a very low-salt, low-fat diet to treat people with severe life-threatening high blood pressure. He found that in a large percentage of severely hypertensive patients this now well-known "rice diet" (*American Journal of Medicine,* 1948; 4:545–77), controlled hypertension. Research at the Pritikin Longevity Center in Santa Monica demonstrated that over 80 percent of people with mild to moderate high blood pressure could be taken off their medication and have their blood pressure controlled by diet alone (*Journal of Cardiac Rehabilitation,* 1983; 3:839-46).

Most people taking diuretics, beta-blockers, and other drugs to control their blood pressure will need to have their dosages reduced when they begin this program. By the end of the first month most will no longer need these drugs to control their blood pressure as long as they continue the grazing lifestyle. As with diabetes medication, *antihypertensive drugs should be reduced or eliminated with the guidance of your physician.*

GOUT

Gout results from excessive levels of uric acid in the blood. Again the rich, highly processed American diet with all its purine-rich meat is a contributing factor. Purines are converted to uric acid in the body. Alcohol reduces the body's ability to get rid of the uric acid, so it is wise not to drink if you are troubled by gout. By adopting the L.A. Diet, many gout sufferers will be able to keep their uric acid levels in the safe range without drugs.

MINOR SYMPTOMS THAT MAY RESULT FROM ADOPTING THIS PROGRAM

While the L.A. Diet Program may do wonders for your health as well as help you permanently get rid of excess body fat, it may produce a few annoying symptoms. Each of the following is a normal and natural consequence of adopting this diet and exercise program.

DELAYED MUSCLE SORENESS

Most people will experience a significant amount of muscle soreness and stiffness when they start a new exercise program. This soreness usually peaks 48 hours after using the muscles in a fashion to which you are unaccustomed. Within a week you should be completely back to normal. This problem can be minimized by starting slowly and stretching after you exercise. If you are a little overambitious on your first long walk in ages, you will likely regret it two days later. Don't let this temporary pain discourage you. As long as you exercise regularly, it will not return unless you stop exercising for two weeks or more.

CAFFEINE WITHDRAWAL

The L.A. Diet calls for the elimination of all unnecessary drugs. Many people experience a rather nasty headache when they stop drinking coffee, tea, and soft drinks and eating chocolate because these are the primary sources of caffeine in the American diet. Headaches from caffeine withdrawal rarely last more than a day or two. You may also feel a little irritable and/or fatigued for the first few days without caffeine, but after that you should be sleeping better, be less irritable, and get fewer headaches.

FLATULENCE

What they say about beans is true. In fact, all high-fiber foods have some tendency to increase intestinal gas. Beans, cabbage, broccoli, cauliflower, brussels sprouts, and turnips are among the worst offenders. Eating smaller but more frequent meals usually reduces this problem. If it occasionally gets out of hand, there is a safe OTC medication that is very effective for reducing intestinal gas. Ask your pharmacist about activated charcoal capsules. The charcoal is not absorbed, but it may reduce the absorption of other medications, so it's best to check with your doctor and/or pharmacist before using charcoal to control intestinal gas, if you are taking a prescription medication by mouth.

GETTING STARTED ON THE RIGHT FOOT

Now you know what to expect from this diet and exercise plan. You've already learned why fat makes you fat and why whatever warms you up slims you down. You now understand why the L.A. Diet Program is the only way to keep the fat off without constantly counting calories and being hungry and fatigued much of the time. But knowing what to expect and why this program is the only safe and effective way to permanently get rid of excess body fat is just the beginning. What follows in the second part of this book is everything you need to know about how to adopt the L.A. Diet. It won't be easy, but the weight loss and improved health and sense of well-being that can result are well worth your efforts.

II
THE L.A. DIET
PROGRAM

by Diane M. Grabowski, M.N.S., R.D.

The L.A. Diet Program works—there is no doubt about it. It works for individual people with individual lifestyles. Eating right to promote a healthy lifestyle requires choice, change, and commitment. Gratification in achieving your ideal body weight and radiating a healthier image are but two of the benefits that can be derived from adopting the L.A. Diet Program's grazing lifestyle.

Why another reducing plan? In response to the never-ending demand for quick and easy weight-loss regimens, new diets appear in great numbers. In general they fail because "dieters" in time return to their former high-fat, high-calorie eating habits. No permanent changes are made in their dietary lifestyles. In addition, many of the diets are poor in nutritional quality, causing metabolic complications that result in physical dysfunction, irrational eating behaviors, nervousness, dehydration, irritability, lethargy, and even death in some cases.

The L.A. Diet Program is not just another reducing plan. It is an answer to the "no win" game many overweight and obese individuals have fallen prey to in an effort to fight the battle of the bulge. It can assist you in breaking away from the dieter's mentality, the deprivation of counting and restricting calories, and the endless game-playing with food and the scale.

Don't wait until Monday to start your new L.A. Diet Program. This is not a diet which you start every other week. Rather, it is a lifestyle plan designed to give you optimal nutrition, health, and overall well-being. Based on a low-fat, low-cholesterol, and high-complex-carbohydrate eating plan, the L.A. Diet Program is nutritious, safe, and well balanced, providing all of the body's nutritional needs.

In the previous chapters, we've discussed the principles and philosophies of the L.A. Diet Program. Now we will provide you with the practical information on how to graze. The chapters ahead will discuss the tools, guidelines, and steps necessary to incorporate grazing into a lifestyle plan. In the first chapter of this section, we will help you get started with your new way of life.

9
GETTING WITH THE
PROGRAM: THE GAME PLAN

How do you translate a low-fat, low-cholesterol, and high-complex-carbohydrate eating program into everyday food choices? What is a carbohydrate? What foods contain fat and cholesterol? How do you know when you're eating too much salt or sugar? Getting the answers to these questions is part of learning about nutrition and being aware of the food choices you're making. Most people don't realize that a piece of cheese or an avocado is 70 to 80 percent fat or that one egg yolk contains close to 300 milligrams of cholesterol for a mere 80 calories. Effective changes in dietary lifestyle begin with knowledge and understanding. We'll start by reviewing some of the basics of food to help you build your dietary know-how.

WHAT IS A CALORIE?

A calorie is a measurement of heat energy derived from the food you eat. Foods provide you with different amounts of calories depending on what major nutrients they contain. For example, fat is more than twice as caloric (giving you approximately 11 calories per gram) as carbohydrates and proteins are (at 4 calories per gram each). Consequently, foods high in fat, such as butter, cream, cheese, and salad dressings are also high in caloric density. Caloric density is defined as the number of calories contained in a food based on the weight of the food. Foods high in caloric density are generally high in fat. Emphasizing low-caloric-density foods is important for tipping the scale to lose weight. Refer to the Caloric Density Chart for specific foods in this chapter.

WHAT IS CHOLESTEROL?

Cholesterol is a waxy, fatlike substance found only in animal foods such as meats, cheese, butter, organ meats, eggs, and animal fats such as lard and tallow. Cholesterol is needed by our bodies to form cell membranes, vitamin D, various hormones, and bile acids. However, the body can produce all of the cholesterol that it needs for these necessary functions. Too much cholesterol taken in the diet is one of the leading causes of heart disease. Vegetables, grains, fruits, and legumes are nonanimal foods that contain no cholesterol.

Cholesterol cannot be burned as a fuel source and therefore must be reduced in the diet to prevent excess buildup. In the L.A. Diet Program, we recommend that you keep your dietary cholesterol low in order to minimize the risk of cardiovascular disease. To reduce your intake of cholesterol, avoid foods high in cholesterol as well as foods high in saturated fat, which can raise the blood cholesterol level. These foods include egg yolks (the egg white is cholesterol-free), organ meats, animal fats such as butter, bacon fat, chicken fat, lard and tallow, cream and cream sauces, hydrogenated or hardened fats or oils, coconut or coconut oil, palm kernel oil, whole milk, and cheeses. Instead, choose animal protein foods such as fish, chicken, turkey, or lean flank or round steak. In addition, limit consumption to approximately 3 to 4 ounces a day. Vegetables, grains, fruits, and legumes are foods of plant origin that contain no cholesterol and should comprise the majority of your diet.

WHAT IS FAT?

Fats fall into two basic categories: saturate fats (solid at room temperature) and unsaturated fats (liquid at room temperature). Unlike cholesterol, fat can be found in both animal and vegetable food sources. For example, although coconuts, vegetable oils, and peanut butter contain no cholesterol, they're all approximately 70–100 percent fat. Other sources of fat include mayonnaise, salad dressings, eggs, meats, cheese, nuts, seeds, lecithin, mono- and diglycerides, margarine, and butter. All added fats are best avoided. This is not to say that fat is not important in your diet. Fat is essential for providing insulation to vital organs, transporting fat-soluble vitamins, and providing the body with the essential fatty acids. However, most whole natural foods contain fat in small but sufficient amounts. In the L.A. Program, we recommend obtaining the fat you need from that found naturally in the foods you eat. Most Americans on the average consume 40 percent of their calories in fat. According to Dr. Kenney's theory, this is the primary reason there is a high incidence of obesity in our country today.

WHAT ARE CARBOHYDRATES?

Carbohydrates are the body's preferred energy source, providing glucose to the brain and other tissues. Carbohydrates are comprised of simple sugars such as honey, table sugar, syrups, and other sweeteners and unrefined complex carbohydrates such as breads, pasta, grains, beans, peas, and starch-based vegetables (e.g., potatoes, yams, squash, and corn). The L.A. Diet Program emphasizes unrefined carbohydrates with simple sugars coming primarily from fruit.

Contrary to popular belief, complex carbohydrates are not fattening. Only 1 percent of the calories in a baked potato are in the form of fat. Unfortunately, most people believe that to lose weight they have to cut out the starches. If we ate more of the starch-based foods and avoided the "fattening" toppings such as butter, sour cream, and rich cream-based sauces, we would most probably be a very lean, thin, and healthy society.

WHAT IS SODIUM?

Salt contains sodium, which is essential to regulating water balance and assisting the blood vessels to maintain proper blood volume. Although essential, too much sodium is dangerous and is linked with hypertension and edema. Most Americans eat too much sodium without realizing it. It is important to remember that sodium is found not only in salt but also in fast foods, prepared products, and canned and frozen goods.

How much sodium do we need? The L.A. Diet Program's general recommendation is 1 milligram of sodium per calorie, not to exceed 1,600 milligrams per day. For example, if the nutritional label on a specific food indicated that there were 80 calories per serving and 240 milligrams of sodium, you would want to avoid this product as it contains more sodium than recommended. It is important to read the labels on the food products you buy and avoid those with too much salt.

WHAT IS PROTEIN?

Protein is an essential nutrient needed to help form new tissues and rebuild old ones. It is an important constituent in every cell of your body. However, most Americans eat over 100 grams of protein per day, which is more than recommended for pregnant women, who generally have elevated needs for all nutrients.

Protein can be found in all natural foods. Best sources include beans, peas, nonfat or skim dairy products, and lean animal protein foods such as fish, poultry, and lean meats. Whole grains and certain vegetables such as asparagus also contribute protein to the diet. By eating a wide variety of foods on the L.A. Diet Program, you'll find it quite easy to get enough protein to meet your requirements.

CALORIC DENSITY

What if someone told you that you could eat as much as you want and still lose weight? And better yet, that you could go all day without feeling hungry or deprived? Well, that's what the L.A. Diet Program can offer those who wish to lose weight, once and for all. How is this possible?

The key to losing weight and keeping it off is to change the composition of your diet from high-fat to high-complex-carbohydrate foods, thus reducing the *caloric density*.

As previously described, caloric density is defined as the number of calories measured for a food based on the weight of the food. Foods vary in their caloric density. For an example of this concept, let's look at the difference between butter and vegetables:

One pound of vegetable oil contains more than 4,000 calories. One pound of vegetables represents a mere 100 calories. Therefore, corn oil is 40 times more calorically dense than vegetables based on an equal weight measure. To lose weight effectively, it would make sense to choose foods with low caloric density. These foods can be eaten in generous portions but will not contain excessive fat and calories. Hunger is not a factor on the L.A. Diet Program. Eating foods low in caloric density throughout the day—eating vegetables, soups, salads, and fruit, helps to fill you up and keep you satisfied.

The following list gives the caloric density of many foods. They are listed in alphabetical order grouped into several levels of caloric density to make it easy to identify the best choices for weight loss. Those in italics are recipes that are included in Part III. An asterisk indicates a food not included in the L.A. Diet Program.

VERY LOW CALORIC DENSITY
(LESS THAN 50 CALORIES PER 100 GRAMS OR 3½ OUNCES)

*Alberto's Italian Eggplant
  Casserole*....................42
Alfalfa sprouts, raw..............41
Apple juice, unsweetened..........47
Applesauced Yogurt, Chilled.......47
Artichokes, canned (without oil).....44
Asparagus.......................20
Basic Chicken Stock, defatted......10
Basic Green Garden Salad.........48
Basic Sparkling Fruit Drink........18
Basic White Sauce..............47
Bean sprouts, mung, raw..........35
Beets, cooked...................32

Bell peppers (red, green, or yellow),
  raw..........................22
Black Bean Soup (chef's version)....32
Bok choy, raw...................24
Broccoli, cooked.................26
Broccoli Pasta Salad.............41
Cabbage, Chinese, cooked.........10
Cantaloupe, fresh................32
Carrot Soup....................26
Carrots, raw....................42
Cauliflower, cooked..............22
Celery, raw.....................16
Celery Root Celeste..............46

LOW CALORIC DENSITY
(50–100 CALORIES PER 100 GRAMS OR 3½ OUNCES)

Apples............................59
Applesauce, unsweetened...........75
Baked Halibut and Peppers.........75
Balsamic Potato Salad............59
Banana Cream Cheese............72
Bananas........................92
Basic Creamy Salad Dressing.......66
Basic Crepe.....................88
Basic Glaze.....................64
Basic Grazing Cream Cheese.......68
Basic Grazing Sour Cream........68
Basic Yogurt Cheese.............56
Black Bean Soup.................66
Blackberries, fresh.................51
Blueberry-Pineapple Topping........56
Blueberries, fresh.................57
Boysenberries, frozen..............50
Cherries, sweet, fresh..............72
Chicken and Vegetables............66
Chili-Orange Sauce (served with
  Pasta and Steamed Vegetables)....87
Chilled Brown Rice Delight........86
Chilled Vegetable Rice Salad.......86
Clams, canned, meat only.........80
Clams Linguini..................90
Corn, frozen....................100
Crab, steamed...................93
Cranberry Relish.................58
Creamy Italian Dressing...........53
Creamy Pasta Primavera...........80
Crunchy Rice Pilaf...............61
Delicious Fruit Crepes.............72
Dill-Yogurt Cheese Spread........53
Early Morning Oatmeal............62
Egg whites, raw..................51
Figs, fresh......................74
Fruit Smoothie..................56
Fruit Sorbet....................88
Ginger Sauce (served with Pasta and
  Steamed Vegetables).............92
Grapes, seedless..................63

Hominy, white, canned............56
Hot Curried Chicken Salad........67
Hot Orange Cinnamon Tea.........66
Kiwifruit, raw....................60
Kumquats, raw...................63
Leeks, raw......................52
Lychees, raw....................66
Mixed vegetables, frozen...........59
Mussels, canned, meat only........95
No-Bake Strawberry Pie...........81
Oatmeal, cooked.................55
Onion-Yogurt Cheese Spread.......68
Oysters, raw.....................66
Parsnips, cooked.................66
Passion fruit, fresh...............100
Pears, fresh.....................50
Peas, green, cooked...............71
Pineapple Chicken................88
Pineapple, fresh..................50
Pineapple Salad for One..........66
Pineapple Yogurt Cheese..........53
Plums, fresh.....................54
Poached Cinnamon Pears..........55
Potatoes, baked..................95
Potatoes, boiled..................76
Potato-Broccoli Soup.............53
Quick and Easy Pizzas............78
Quick Corn Chowder.............62
Raspberries, fresh.................50
Salmon Salad...................75
Savory Cream Cheese.............84
Sherry Garlic Dressing............60
Snow peas, fresh or frozen, raw......53
Spaghetti.......................67
Spicy Spanish Rice...............77
Spinach Cheese..................52
Summer Salad...................56
Sunny Morning Potatoes..........65
Sunshine Fruit and Yogurt Salad....70
Supreme Garden Salad............71
Sweet 'n' Sour Carrot Salad........68

Tasty Fruit and Rice..............99
Teriyaki Sauce...................67
Thousand Island Dressing........66
Tomato-Caper Sauce (served with
   Pasta and Steamed Vegetables)....66
Tomato Rice Salad..............71

Vegetables and Beef Oriental Style...69
Water chestnuts, canned...........80
Yam Salad Deluxe................75
Yam Stew Deluxe................75
Yogurt Freeze...................51

MODERATE CALORIC DENSITY
(100–200 CALORIES PER 100 GRAMS OR 3½ OUNCES)

Basic Brown Rice...............106
Basic Spice Cake...............140
Bean and Rice Soft Tacos........117
Beans, white, cooked.............118
Black-eyed peas, cooked..........108
Bluefish, broiled.................157
Butter beans, frozen.............145
Cheesecake with Fruit Topping.....107
Chestnuts, raw, fresh.............194
Chicken, white meat, cooked.......166
Cod, broiled....................170
Corn Bread....................170
Date and Raisin Cream Cheese....111
Dr. Jay's Blueberry Oat Bran
   Muffins......................166
Everyday Bran Muffins..........180
Flank Steak, cooked.............196
French Toast...................105
Garbanzo beans, cooked..........179
Haddock, cooked................141
Halibut, cooked.................171
Hen, cooked, without skin.........180
Kidney beans, cooked............118
Lentils, cooked..................106

Lima beans, cooked..............138
Oatmeal Pancakes...............143
Orange and Banana Cake.........184
Orange Roughy in Lime and Ginger
   Sauce........................108
Pasta, cooked...................147
Persimmons, raw................128
Poached Salmon with Vegetables...129
Prunes, dried, cooked.............107
Quick Spicy Chicken.............141
Rice, brown, long-grain, cooked....118
Salmon, cooked.................182
Scallops, cooked.................112
Sherry-Garlic Dressing...........107
Shrimp, cooked.................116
Snow Pea and Pasta Salad........108
Spice Cake....................138
Split peas, cooked...............115
Soy beans, cooked..............130
Sweet potatoes, baked...........141
Swordfish, cooked...............174
Trout, cooked...................196
Tuna, white meat, water-packed....128
Turkey, white meat, cooked........176

MODERATELY HIGH CALORIC DENSITY
(200–400 CALORIES PER 100 GRAMS OR 3½ OUNCES)

Apricots, dried..................237
Bagels, water...................296
Bass, striped, broiled.............228
Bread, rye.....................264
Bread, whole wheat..............244
*Coconut, fresh.................346

Currants, dried..................283
Dates, dried....................274
*Egg yolks, raw.................348
English muffins.................236
Figs, dried.....................255
*Honey........................306

Hortensia's Rice Crispy Squares....248

*Jams and jellies, with sugar.......275

Kingfish, cooked...............255

Lychees, dried.................277

Mackerel, broiled..............230

Popcorn, popped, plain..........386

Prunes, dried...................239

Raisins, dried..................302

Sea bass, cooked...............228

*Vodka.......................274

Yeast, dry active...............288

HIGH CALORIC DENSITY
(400–650 CALORIES PER 100 GRAMS OR 3½ OUNCES)

*Almonds.....................598

*Beef rib, entire, cooked.........440

*Blue cheese salad dressing.......504

*Cashews.....................561

*Chocolate, sweet...............529

*Filbert nuts...................634

*Peanuts.....................564

*Peanut butter..................580

*Potato chips...................567

*Salami.......................450

*Sesame seeds..................580

*Sirloin steak...................408

*Sunflower seeds...............560

VERY HIGH CALORIC DENSITY
(650–900 CALORIES PER 100 GRAMS OR 3½ OUNCES)

*Brazil nuts...................654

*Butter.......................720

*Coconut, dried, unsweetened......662

*Macadamia nuts...............691

*Margarine....................720

*Mayonnaise...................697

*Pecans.......................687

*Salad oils.....................884

*Shortenings...................900

10
BALANCING THE
GRAZING ACT

Grazing sensibly means choosing a variety of foods in order to obtain sufficient nutrients to provide a well-balanced diet. Too often people who want to lose weight fall prey to fad diets that advocate eating one type of food or eliminating others. This can be dangerous to their nutritional status and at the same time cause them to develop irrational eating habits.

Almost everyone has heard of a "balanced diet." However, not everyone knows what this means. It's probably safe to say that a "balanced" diet is one that promotes or, at least, is compatible with optimal health. However, in obtaining a "balanced" diet, it's just as important to avoid dietary excesses as it is to avoid dietary deficiencies. In other words, the danger of consuming too much fat, cholesterol, sugar, salt, and alcohol is as equally significant as eating enough fruits, vegetables, nonfat dairy products, lean animal products, and whole grains. Let's look at some specific guidelines to assure that you'll satisfy your nutritional requirements while still deriving the benefits of the L.A. Diet Program.

GENERAL GUIDELINES FOR
GRAZING YOUR WAY TO HEALTH

1. Eat a variety of foods each day. Use the following guide to
   assist you in selecting from each of the five food groups:
   - Dairy (nonfat): 2 servings per day
   - Vegetables: 10 or more servings per day
   - Fruits: 3 or more servings per day
   - Breads, grains, and cereals: 4 or more servings per day
   - High-protein foods: 3–4 ounces lean animal protein foods
     per day or 3–4 ounces of high-protein vegetable foods per
     day

   To understand what constitutes a serving, refer to the
   section following these guidelines. The recommended
   servings listed above provide approximately 1,200 calories. However, it's not important to count calories. Rather,
   focus on eating the serving allotments from each of the
   food groups. Do *not* eat fewer than the number of servings
   indicated.

2. Include 2 daily servings from the dairy group which provides a good source of riboflavin, calcium, and vitamin D.
   The recommended intake is limited to prevent obtaining
   too much protein in your diet.

3. In the high-protein category, limit intake to 3–4 ounces
   per day for maximum weight loss and to control intake of
   protein, fat, and cholesterol.

4. For maximum weight loss, vegetables can be eaten in
   unlimited amounts. Eat plenty of raw and cooked vegetables daily for snacks or with meals, which provide valuable nutrients with very few calories—perfect grazing
   food. Also, foods with a low caloric density should be
   emphasized in order to help you "fill" up without consuming too many calories. (Refer to the Caloric Density
   chart in Chapter 9.)

5. For those who wish to maintain *or* gain weight, whole
   grains, fruits, and vegetables can be eaten in greater
   quantity.

6. If consuming 1,500 calories or more, choose up to 5 ounces of high-protein foods, but no more than 3–4 ounces as lean animal protein. If consuming 2,500 calories or more, choose up to 7 ounces of high-protein foods, with only half in the form of lean animal protein.

7. If you choose not to drink or eat dairy products, an additional 4 ounces of high-protein vegetable foods such as $\frac{1}{2}$ cup of cooked beans or 6 ounces of tofu can be included. However, do not include extra animal protein such as chicken, fish, or turkey. Also, choose two additional servings of dark green vegetables such as kale, collards, broccoli, or romaine lettuce to provide additional calcium.

8. Include breakfast on a regular basis, especially if trying to lose weight. Breakfast provides valuable nutrients and refuels the body after the previous hours of fasting. Hot cereals are a good choice and tend to be more satisfying than cold cereals.

Remember to get exercise on a regular basis. Besides improving your health and weight-loss program, exercise gives you a feeling of well-being and puts you in the right frame of mind for sensible eating.

SERVINGS OF FOODS IN THE FIVE FOOD GROUPS

The following chart provides a list of foods suggested for the L.A. Diet Program. Use this guide to choose foods in the appropriate amounts as recommended, for planning meals and snacks.

Dairy Foods

Recommended servings: 2 per day
Each serving provides 80 calories, 12 g carbohydrate, 8 g protein, trace fat, 4 mg cholesterol
Skim or nonfat milk..........8 ounces
Skim or nonfat yogurt........6 ounces

1% fat or less buttermilk......8 ounces   *1% low-fat cottage cheese....2 ounces
*Nonfat dry-curd cottage cheese......2   Nonfat dry powdered milk.......⅓ cup
   ounces   Evaporated skim milk........4 ounces

---

*If low-sodium brand cannot be obtained, limit consumption to 1 serving per day
due to a lower calcium and higher sodium content.

Vegetables (Low Starch Content)

Recommended servings: 10 or more per day
One serving is 1 cup of raw vegetables or ½ cup cooked
Each serving provides 25 calories, 6 g carbohydrate, 2 g protein, trace fat,
   0 cholesterol

Alfalfa sprouts
Artichokes, fresh or canned in water
   (rinsed and drained)
Asparagus
Bamboo shoots
Bean sprouts, mung
Beans, green or yellow, wax or string
Beet greens, raw
Beets, fresh or canned (packed in own
   juice)
Bok choy
Breadfruit (¼ cup)
Broccoli
Brussels sprouts
Cabbage, all varieties
Carrots
Celery
Celery root, fresh or canned (rinsed and
   drained)
Cilantro (fresh coriander leaves)
Chayote
Chicory
Chilies
Chinese cabbage
Chives
Collard greens
Cucumber
Eggplant
Endive
Escarole

Fennel leaves
Garden cress
Garlic
Gingerroot
Green beans, French style
Green beans, snap
Jerusalem artichokes
Kale
Kohlrabi
Leeks
Lettuce, all varieties
Mushrooms
Mustard greens
Mustard spinach
Okra
Onions, all varieties
Parsley
Parsnips
Peppers, bell
Pimientos
Radishes
Rhubarb
Rutabaga
Sauerkraut, canned (rinsed and drained)
Scallions
Shallots
Snow peas, Chinese
Soybean sprouts
Spinach
Squash, summer

Tomatoes, fresh
Tomato juice
Turnips

Turnip greens
Zucchini

Fruits

Recommended servings: 3 or more per day
Each serving provides 60 calories, 10 g carbohydrate, trace protein, trace fat,
  0 cholesterol

Acerola, raw.................1 cup
Apple...................1 medium
Apple juice, concentrate...2 tablespoons
Apple juice, unsweetened........⅓ cup
Applesauce, unsweetened........½ cup
Apricots, dried..............8 halves
Apricots, raw..............4 medium
Bananas, raw..............½ medium
Blackberries, frozen, unsweetened ½ cup
Blackberries, raw..............1 cup
Blueberries, frozen, unsweetened.. ½ cup
Blueberries, raw...............¾ cup
Boysenberries, frozen, unsweetened
  ....½ cup
Cantaloupe, raw.. 1 cup pieces or ¼ slice
Carambola, raw (star fruit)...1 medium
Casaba melon, raw........1 cup pieces
Cherimoya, raw...........¹⁄₁₀ medium
Cherries, canned (water packed).. ½ cup
Cherries, sweet, raw..........10 each
Crab apples, raw...............¾ cup
Cranberries, raw...............1 cup
Currants, dried.. 2 tablespoons or ⅛ cup
Dates, dried...............3 medium
Figs, dried................1 medium
Figs, raw.................2 medium
Fruit cocktail, packed in water... ½ cup
Grapefruit, raw (pink or white)
  ....½ medium
Grapes, raw (Thompson seedless)
  ....15 small
Guava, raw...............1 medium
Honeydew melon......1 cup or ¼ slice
Kiwifruit, raw.............1 medium

Kumquats, raw............5 medium
Lemons, raw.............3 medium
Loquats, raw.............10 medium
Lychees, dried................⅛ cup
Lychees, raw.............10 medium
Mandarin oranges, water-packed
  ....½ cup
Mangoes, raw.............½ medium
Nectarines, raw............1 medium
Orange juice concentrate.. 2 tablespoons
Orange juice, unsweetened.......½ cup
Oranges, navel, raw.........1 medium
Papayas, raw..............½ medium
Passion fruit, raw...........3 medium
Peaches, canned, water-packed....1 cup
Peaches, dried..............2 halves
Peaches, raw..............2 medium
Pears, canned, water-packed......1 cup
Pear, raw...................1 small
Persimmons, raw...........2 medium
Pineapple, canned, unsweetened... ⅓ cup
Pineapple juice...............½ cup
Pineapple, raw...........1 cup, pieces
Plums, raw...............2 medium
Pomegranates, raw.........½ medium
Prune juice...................⅓ cup
Prunes, dried..............3 medium
Raisins, all varieties......2 tablespoons
Raspberries, raw...............1 cup
Strawberries, raw..............1 cup
Tangelos, raw................2 small
Tangerines, raw..............2 small
Watermelon, raw...............1 cup

Starches (Breads, Grains, and Related Foods)

Recommended servings: 4 or more per day
Each serving provides 80 calories, 12 g carbohydrate, 2 g protein, 1 g fat,
  0 cholesterol

BREADS, CRACKERS, AND RELATED FOODS

Bagels, water.............¹/₂ medium
Bread, whole wheat, rye,
  pumpernickel...............1 slice
Breadsticks.................4 regular
Bun, whole wheat, hamburger or hot
  dog......................¹/₂ regular
English muffin, whole wheat..¹/₂ regular
Matzo crackers, plain.........³/₄ ounce

Melba toast, whole wheat.......5 slices
Pancakes, whole wheat 1 4-inch-diameter
Pita bread, whole wheat 1 6-inch pocket
Popcorn, no oil or butter 3 cups popped
Rolls, whole wheat, sourdough or
  French...........1 2-inch-diameter
Rye crisp crackers, unseasoned.......4
Tortillas, corn........1 6-inch-diameter

STARCHY VEGETABLES

Corn, fresh, on the cob, cooked
  ....1 4-inch ear
Corn, fresh or frozen, kernels,
  cooked...................¹/₂ cup
Hominy, cooked...............¹/₂ cup
Parsnips............²/₃ cup or 1 small
Peas, green, cooked...........¹/₂ cup

Potatoes, baked or boiled....1 medium
Potatoes, mashed.............¹/₂ cup
Pumpkin, canned or fresh, cooked ³/₄ cup
Squash, winter (acorn, butternut,
  banana).............³/₄ cup cooked
Sweet potatoes, baked ¹/₃ cup or ¹/₂ small
Yams, baked.........¹/₃ cup or ¹/₂ small

FLOURS, GRAINS, CEREALS, AND PASTAS

Arrowroot.............2 tablespoons
Barley, cooked................¹/₂ cup
Bran, unprocessed, raw..........¹/₂ cup
Buckwheat flour........3 tablespoons
Cereal, cold (without sugar or oils)
  ....³/₄ cup
Cereal, hot (any whole grain)....¹/₂ cup
Cornmeal, cooked........3 tablespoons
Cornstarch............2 tablespoons
Cracked wheat (bulgur), cooked..¹/₂ cup
Cream of Wheat (farina), cooked ¹/₂ cup
Grapenuts cereal...............¹/₄ cup
Grits, cooked................¹/₂ cup
Kasha (buckwheat groats), cooked ¹/₃ cup
Macaroni, whole wheat, cooked...¹/₂ cup

Matzo meal.............3 tablespoons
Noodles, rice, cooked...........¹/₂ cup
Noodles, whole wheat (eggless),
  cooked...................¹/₂ cup
Oat bran, raw.................¹/₂ cup
Oatmeal, cooked...............¹/₂ cup
Pasta, whole wheat or enriched,
  cooked...................¹/₂ cup
Potato flour...........2¹/₂ tablespoons
Rice flour.............3 tablespoons
Rice, long-grain, brown, cooked..¹/₂ cup
Rice, short-grain, brown, cooked..¹/₂ cup
Rice, wild, cooked.............¹/₂ cup
Rye cereal, cooked.............¹/₂ cup
Rye flour...............4 tablespoons

Shredded Wheat cereal
............½ cup or 1 large biscuit
Steel-cut oats, cooked...........½ cup

Wheatena, cooked.............½ cup
Whole wheat flour.......3 tablespoons

High-Protein Foods

Recommended servings:

For maxium weight loss: 3–4 ounces per day of lean animal protein (maximum) or
3–4 ounces of vegetable protein

For intake of 1,500 calories or more: up to 5 ounces of high-protein foods, but only
3–4 ounces in the form of lean animal protein

For intake of 2,500 calories or more: up to 7 ounces of high-protein foods, but only
3–4 ounces in the form of lean animal protein

One serving is 3½ ounces or 100 grams cooked food.

FISH AND SHELLFISH

One ounce provides 35 calories, 0 carbohydrate, 7 g protein, 7 g fat, 20 mg
cholesterol

Fish, all lean varieties, cooked (cod,
flounder, haddock, halibut, perch,
pike, seabass, red snapper, sole,
sturgeon, swordfish, trout, tuna)
(water-packed)...........3½ ounces

Mollusks (abalone, clams, mussels,
oysters, scallops) (cooked)..3½ ounces
*Crustaceans (crab, lobster, shrimp,
crayfish, raw............3½ ounces

*Crustaceans contain twice as much cholesterol per ounce as other fish choices.

POULTRY, FATTIER FISH, AND LEAN MEAT

One ounce provides 55 calories, 0 carbohydrate, 7 g protein, 7 g fat, 25 mg
cholesterol

Chicken, breast, white meat,
cooked................3½ ounces
Turkey, breast, white meat,
cooked................3½ ounces

Fish, cooked: carp, catfish, mackerel,
mullet, salmon, whitefish, fresh
tuna..................3½ ounces
Flank steak, cooked........3½ ounces
Round steak, cooked.......3½ ounces

VEGETABLE PROTEIN (LEGUMES)

The following foods yield 3–4 ounces from the vegetable protein group.

Each serving provides approximately 80 calories, 7 g protein, 21 g carbohydrate, trace fat, 0 cholesterol

Beans, dried, cooked, all varieties ⅓ cup

Beans, lima, fresh..............½ cup

Black-eyed peas (cow peas), cooked...................½ cup

Lentils, cooked................⅓ cup

Peas, dried, cooked............⅓ cup

*Tofu (soybean curd), raw.....4 ounces

---

*Tofu and soybeans have a substantially lower carbohydrate content (2.7 grams per 4 ounces) and a higher fat content (4.8 grams per 4 ounces) than other legumes.

11
SETTING UP A
WINNING KITCHEN

Out with the old, in with the new. This cliché certainly carries truth when changing your old kitchen into a new grazing arena. A healthier way of eating requires you to keep a well-stocked kitchen, which is a fundamental part of making your cooking simple and successful. Also, having on hand only the proper products and ingredients makes it easy to avoid old habits. If gorging foods are still sitting on the shelf, you'll be tempted to return to former ways of eating. Don't save a bag of chips or a box of cookies for the grandchildren or unexpected company. Rather, fill the cupboards with healthier snack options. Out of sight, out of mind! Grandchildren, friends, and relatives can benefit from eating nutritious snacks such as popcorn, fresh fruit, and delicious desserts prepared without fat, sugar, or salt.

Cleaning out the cupboards, restocking the pantry, and filling the refrigerator with grazing foods are the first steps to making your new L.A. Diet Program a successful one. Let's begin with the basic equipment needed for starting out on the right foot.

EQUIPMENT

Streamline your kitchen as much as possible. There's no need to buy extra gadgets or supplies that have little purpose. Instead, focus on the essentials that will be used frequently and in several ways. Here's a list that can assist you in setting up your kitchen. Please note, however, that many of the items are optional. You can start the Grazing Program with as little as a skillet, spoon, fork, and knife!

Pots and Pans

Stainless-steel pots and pans: skillets, various-sized saucepans, large stockpots.
Nonstick skillets
Nonstick muffin pan
Nonstick cookie sheet

Nonstick loaf pan
Nonstick cake pans, round
Nonstick casserole pans (rectangular or square)
Nonstick wok
Nonstick crepe pan

Motor Equipment

Food processor (with a direct drive motor for more power)
Blender
Electric hand-mixer

Crock pot
Pressure cooker
Air-popper (for popcorn, optional)
Microwave oven (optional)

Small Kitchen Appliances and Tools

Steamer (folding or collapsible style)
Canisters (for storing grains, dried legumes, etc.)
Airtight sealed containers (various sizes for storage)
Freezer bags
Wire racks
Garlic press
Pastry brush
Egg separator (optional)
Chopping board
Knives (a good set for slicing and chopping; various sizes)
Colander

Strainer
Ice cube trays (for freezing chicken broth, fruit juices, etc.)
Wire whisks (large and small)
Mixing bowls
Grater
Vegetable peeler
Scale
Sifter
Ladles
Measuring cups
Measuring spoons
Rolling pin

STOCKING YOUR HERB AND SPICE SHELF

Herbs

The use of herbs in cooking is a culinary tradition in every cuisine. For flavoring and garnishing, their use can increase the palatability and eye appeal of any recipe. Fresh herbs are always preferred to dried ones, and many can be grown at home in small pots. To store fresh herbs, wrap in paper towels, place in plastic bags, and store in the vegetable compartment of the refrigerator or trim the stems, place in cups of water (like flowers), and place in the refrigerator.

Dried herbs are much more concentrated than fresh because the water has been removed. For every teaspoon of dried herbs, use one tablespoon of fresh herbs. Store dried herbs in airtight sealed containers in a cool, dry place. Label with name and date. Keep for up to six months.

Herbs can also be frozen, although they will not have the same quality as fresh herbs. One method is to spread the leaves on a cookie sheet and place in a freezer; then store in freezer bags.

Basil	Marjoram/sweet marjoram
Bay leaves	Mint
Celery seed	Oregano
Chervil	Parsley
Chives	Rosemary
Cilantro leaves (coriander)	Sage
Curry leaf	Savory
Dill	Tarragon
Fennel	Thyme
Fenugreek	

Spices and Seeds

Spices today are used widely in the kitchen to flavor and season foods. Spices can be found in both fresh and dried forms. To store spices, keep in airtight sealed containers and place in a cool, dry area. Spices can be refrigerated to help them retain flavor and freshness.

Allspice	Cayenne pepper
Anise	Chili powder
Annatto	Chinese five-spice powder
Caraway	Cinnamon
Cardamom	Cloves

Coriander
Cumin
Fenugreek, seeds
Garlic powder
Ginger
Horseradish
Mace
Nutmeg

Onion powder
Paprika
Pepper, black or white
Poppy seeds
Saffron
Sesame seeds (for garnishing)
Turmeric

PANTRY LIST

Dry Storage

CANNED AND BOTTLED GOODS

Applesauce, unsweetened
Artichoke hearts (water-packed)
Beans (preferably without sugar)
Beets (packed in own juice)
Chilies, green
Extracts, pure
Fruits (packed in own juice): fruit cocktail, peaches, pears, pineapple
Milk, evaporated skim
Mustard, Dijon (unsalted)
Nonstick cooking spray (e.g., Pam)
Pimientos, sliced or chopped (water-packed)
Pumpkin
Salmon
Salsa, unsalted

Soy sauce, low-sodium
Spaghetti sauce (no added sugar, salt, or oil)
Tomato products; unsalted: crushed tomatoes, whole (peeled) tomatoes, tomato sauce, tomato juice, tomato puree, tomato paste, plum tomatoes, stewed tomatoes
Tuna (water-packed), preferably unsalted
Vinegars: rice vinegar (unsweetened), red wine vinegar, white vinegar, balsamic vinegar, raspberry vinegar, herbal blend vinegars (Paula's)
Water chestnuts
Worcestershire sauce

PACKAGED DRY GOODS

Arrowroot
Baking powder, low-sodium or regular
Baking soda
Beans, peas, and lentils, dried
Carob powder, unsweetened
Cereals: oatmeal, long-grain brown rice, triticale, kasha, buckwheat, bulgur, millet, cornmeal, seven- and four-grain cereals, barley
Cereals, whole grain, cold: Shredded Wheat, Grapenuts, Nutty Rice

Cornstarch
Flour, whole wheat
Flour, whole wheat blend (contains 50% whole wheat and 50% unbleached white), used primarily for making bread
Fruit, dried: apricots, currants, dates, peaches, pears, raisins
Gelatin, unflavored
Herbs and spices, dried (see lists above)
Matzo meal

Nonfat buttermilk powder
Nonfat milk powder
Oat bran
Pasta, whole wheat (all shapes and
  sizes)
Pectin powder

Popcorn
Rice, wild
Tapioca, quick-cooking
Wheat bran
Yeast, rapid-rise

FRESH FOODS

Bread, whole wheat
Chicken breasts (when ready to use)
Eggs (for purpose of using whites)
Fish (when ready to use)
Flank or round steak, lean (when ready
  to use)
Fruit concentrates, liquid form
  (nonfrozen varieties)
Fruit concentrates, unsweetened (allow
  to thaw in a sealed glass jar)
Fruit spreads (without sugar or honey)
Fruit syrups (without sugar or honey)

Herbs and spices, fresh
Onions
Potatoes: sweet potatoes, white
  potatoes, yams
Salad dressings (without oil or salt)
Sauces, dressings, and other recipes
  (homemade or prepared; keep opened
  bottles of various sauces, dressings,
  fruits, etc., in refrigerator)
Squash, winter
Tortillas, corn
Vegetables, cut-up raw (for snacking)

Refrigerator Storage

Buttermilk, 1% or less
Cottage cheese, nonfat dry-curd
Cottage cheese, 1% or less
Fruits, perishable

Garlic, chopped or crushed
Milk, skim or nonfat
Vegetables, perishable
Yogurt, nonfat plain

Freezer Storage

Bread, whole grain (for later use)
Chicken, beef, or fish stock, defatted
Fish, chicken, or meat, frozen (for later
  use)
Fruit juice concentrates, frozen (for later
  use)

Fruits, frozen (without sugar)
Gingerroot, grated fresh
Herbs and spices, fresh
Soups and entrees, prepared
Vegetables, frozen (without salt)

SHOPPING FOR GRAZING FOODS

Use the food lists above to assist you in planning your grocery list.
When changing your dietary lifestyle, it's important to remember that it
may require extra time to shop for new foods, products, and ingredients.

However, with more time spent on the L.A. Diet Program, grocery shopping will become a simple process.

Your shopping may involve going to more than one kind of store. Many of the food products or special ingredients recommended in the Grazing Program can be found in specialty or gourmet shops, local health food stores, or your neighborhood market. Most major grocery chains now carry a special health section containing valuable products that can add variety to your shopping list. In addition, more and more food products are available in low-fat form, so keep your eyes open for new items acceptable to the L.A. Diet Program.

The following are tips to help you when shopping.

1. Read labels carefully. Use the following guidelines to increase your awareness of fat, cholesterol, salt, and sugar. Key words and ingredients to watch out for:

 • Vegetable fat: mono- and diglycerides, lecithin, vegetable oil, partially hydrogenated fats, margarine, shortenings, coconut and palm kernel oil (both contain saturated fat)

 • Animal fat—contains cholesterol and is usually high in saturated fat: cream, lard, tallow, chicken fat or schmaltz, beef fat, egg yolks, whole milk, butter, bacon fat, pork fat, salt pork, cheese products, whole-milk solids

 • Salt: table salt (sodium chloride), sodium, baking soda, baking powder, soy sauce, sea salt, seaweeds, miso, monosodium glutamate (MSG), sodium saccharin, sodium nitrates or nitrites, smoked foods, salt-cured foods

 • Refined sugars: any ingredient ending in *ose*; for example, sucrose, fructose, maltose, dextrose, lactose, and glucose; also, honey, corn syrup, high-fructose corn syrup, brown sugar

2. Fat content of a food product should not exceed 15% of the total calories. To determine the percentage of fat, follow this formula:

$9 \times$ grams of fat/total calories $\times 100 =$ _____%

9 represents the calories per 1 gram of fat

Grams of fat and total calories to be determined from a nutritional panel

For example: 1 ounce of cheddar cheese contains 100 calories and 9 grams of fat: $9 \times 9/100 \times 100 = 81\%$

Therefore, 1 ounce of cheddar cheese contains 81% of its total calories in fat, and this food should be avoided.

3. Limit sodium intake to 1,500 milligrams per day. When evaluating food products, choose items that on the average do not exceed 1 milligram of sodium per calorie. In cases when milligrams of sodium slightly exceed calories, use these items in small amounts.

4. To help reduce shopping time, make a grocery list to take with you.

5. Get to know your store managers. Ask them to order special items whenever possible.

6. Locate a reliable health food store in your area. Also, check the gourmet stores for special items.

7. Buy oats, wheat, cornmeal, rice, and other grains in bulk. A variety of grains can be purchased from your local health food store.

8. When buying bread products, be sure they're made with 100 percent stone-ground wheat. Many breads contain "wheat flour," which is a blend of whole wheat and refined white flour.

9. Select a variety of foods. Experiment with exotic fruits, whole grains, and vegetables.

10. Be sure to allow for enough shopping time. Initially it will take longer to shop because you'll be reading labels and looking for new food items. Enjoy the adventure and make it fun!

STORAGE

Storing perishable and nonperishable items properly can enhance both flavor and freshness of your foods. In addition, if you cook food in large quantities, storing the excess can save time and provide easy-to-prepare leftovers. Let's say, for example, you make a large potful of soup. Take half and freeze it. Serve the remainder throughout the week as part of lunch, dinner, or to enjoy as a snack.

Here are a few tips about storing your foods:

• Store uncooked grains such as oats, barley, rice, and wheat in clear canisters for everyday use. If buying in bulk, freeze uncooked grains to preserve freshness and flavor.

- Store fresh herbs and spices in the refrigerator or freezer.
- Store cooked foods in airtight containers or durable plastic bags. You can store foods in individual serving sizes and simply reheat when ready to use. Plastic boiling bags can also be used for storing extras. To reheat, place in boiling water or use a microwave.
- Freeze defatted chicken broth in ice cube trays or Styrofoam egg cartons. After freezing, remove and store in plastic bags. Use as "bouillon cubes." Freeze remainder of broth for up to six months.
- Egg whites can be frozen in ice cube trays or Styrofoam egg cartons. Thaw to room temperature before using.
- Almost all foods can be frozen, such as beans, bean entrees, lasagne, tomato-based recipes, breads, sauces, pancakes, French toast, soups, stews, and casseroles. However, avoid freezing high-water-containing vegetables such as lettuce, tomatoes, celery, and cabbage.
- When preparing pancakes, French toast, or crepes, make extra. Store the remainder by placing each between sheets of wax paper, parchment paper, or freezer paper, then wrap them in plastic and freeze. To reuse, warm in microwave, toaster, or oven.
- Meat, poultry, and fish can be frozen cooked or uncooked. Wrap unused portions in plastic or freezer bags to preserve freshness.

12
YOUR NEW EATING PLAN

Eating throughout the day is an essential component of the L.A. Diet Program. Having six to seven mini-meals a day is not difficult, but it may at first seem nearly impossible to do. This chapter presents guidelines and tips for successfully planning your eating program, whether you wish to lose weight or simply learn how to eat a healthful, well-balanced diet.

It is important to note that the L.A. Diet Program is designed for healthy adults. Although everyone benefits from the basic principles of eating a low-fat, low-cholesterol, high-complex-carbohydrate diet, individuals such as growing children and pregnant or lactating women have special dietary needs and should consult with their physician or registered dietitian for specific nutritional guidelines.

Most people wouldn't think that snacking could be part of a weight loss program. On most diets, snacking is generally considered "cheating." On the L.A. Diet Program, however, snacks are an essential part of your eating plan. Healthy light foods throughout the day can help take the edge off your appetite, stabilize blood sugar, and prevent feelings of weakness or fatigue.

The concept of snacking goes back many years. A form of the mid-afternoon snack originated early in Queen Victoria's reign, with the

Duchess of Bedford, who habitually suffered a "sinking feeling around five o'clock." She started taking tea with thin sandwiches, and the afternoon tea hour was born, a custom that was to evolve ultimately into a serious meal known as "high tea."

A "sinking feeling" is not uncommon among dieters, who by four or five o'clock are reaching for something sweet to help combat the hunger and fatigue that result from their depleted glycogen stores. Those sweets, unfortunately, leave them hungry for more. The added calories, fat, and sugar sabotage both willpower and weight loss.

Rather than give into the never-ending battle with hunger and dieting, change your snacking habits to include healthful between-meal energizers. The key is to choose foods loaded with important nutrients that taste good yet contain few calories. That's what grazing is all about.

Guidelines follow to help you better plan your menus. Ideas and suggestions are listed for breakfast, lunch, dinner, and snacks. Develop a collection of your own favorite meals, foods, and flavorful combinations to tailor the L.A. Diet Program to your lifestyle.

BREAKFAST

Breakfast is the most important meal of the day, especially while you're trying to lose weight. It refuels the body and restores your carbohydrate reserves after 12–14 hours of fasting.

1. Include one or more servings from the complex carbohydrate food group, such as ½ cup hot cooked cereal (oatmeal, rice, cracked wheat, barley, cornmeal) or ¾ cup acceptable cold cereal or 1 slice bread. Hot cereals tend to warm you up, and they satisfy the appetite more than cold cereals.
2. Include a fruit serving with your breakfast. Banana cooked with hot cereal, a fresh fruit cup, or berries with yogurt are tasty fruit options to try.
3. Include a dairy serving such as a cup of skim milk or 6 ounces of plain nonfat yogurt with your meal to provide protein and calcium.
4. Experiment with a variety of breakfast menu options. Avoid eating the same thing every day to prevent bore-

dom. Try some of these breakfast suggestions (italicized dishes are recipes included in Part III):

Egg white omelet
Whole grain pancakes
French toast with fruit topping
Hot cooked cereal with banana and raisins
Yogurt with Grapenuts and fruit
Blueberry Crepes
Water bagel with *Grazing Cream Cheese*
"Veggie bagel": bagel toasted with mustard, onions, sprouts, and tomato slices

Grazing muffins (bran, blueberry, or corn with fresh fruit)
Steamed corn tortillas with salsa and boiled beans
Hot cooked rice with cooked apple
Any left-over grazing dessert; e.g., *No-Bake Strawberry Pie* or *Cheesecake with Fruit Topping*

LUNCH AND DINNER

1. Include unlimited amounts of raw vegetables with your meals. Make creative salads and use a tasty low-fat salad dressing to flavor. Remember, for maximum weight loss, emphasize ample amounts of vegetables.
2. Include at least 2 cups (4 servings) of cooked green, yellow, or orange vegetables with your meals. Vegetables can be served as side dishes or tossed into salads, soups, or casseroles.
3. Include at least one serving from the complex carbohydrate group with both lunch and dinner. Examples include $\frac{1}{2}$ cup whole wheat pasta, brown rice, or other cooked grain, or one slice pita bread or whole wheat roll, or one medium potato.
4. Include a hot bowl of soup before your meal. Remember, hot soups tend to warm you up and satisfy the appetite yet provide few calories. Experiment with the many tasty soup recipes in Part III, Chapter 14.
5. Include one or more servings of fruit as dessert or as an appetizer.
6. If eating animal protein, be sure to limit portions to 3–4 ounces per day or substitute 3–4 ounces from the nonmeat protein sources such as legumes. If you're not trying to lose weight, 6–8 servings of high-protein foods may be

included. However, always limit animal protein to 3–4 ounces per day. (Refer to the five food groups in Chapter 10.)

7. It's important to include a variety of menus for both lunch and dinner. Refer to Part III to help you get started. Here are a few more suggestions (italicized recipes can be found in Part III):

Creative colorful salads using a variety of fresh vegetables

Stuffed pita sandwiches with a bowl of soup

Baked potato with salad and fresh fruit

Chicken Curry with rice and salad

Steamed fish with vegetables and fruit

One-pot dishes filled with plenty of vegetables

Lasagne

Oriental vegetables

Quick and Easy Pizza

Hot soup, *Corn Bread*, and salad

Vegetable chili (create your own by combining vegetables, beans, and tomato or spaghetti sauce)

Creamy Pasta Primavera

Vegetable omelet

Spaghetti

SNACKS

---

1. Include 2–3 snacks each day. A suggested snack schedule: mid-morning (10:00 A.M.), mid-afternoon (3:00 P.M.), and evening (8:00 P.M.). However, there's no need to follow a clock. Snack when feeling hungry, which may vary from individual to individual.

2. Avoid heavy snacks, especially in the evening. Opt for light, low-calorie choices. Snacks simply refuel you enough to normalize your blood sugar and prevent hunger.

3. Avoid skipping snacks to save calories. Remember, snacking is an important part of the L.A. Diet Program.

4. Select snacks that are high in nutritional value. For maximum weight loss, emphasize foods with low caloric density such as vegetables, hot soups, and salads.

   Here are some other suggestions that can be made at home and taken to the office or anywhere else when you'll be away from your kitchen (italicized recipes are included in Part III):

Air-popped popcorn

Raw vegetables with an acceptable dip or salsa

Baked yam or sweet potato with applesauce and cinnamon

Fresh fruit and yogurt

Whole grain crackers and vegetables
Hot vegetable soup
Fresh fruit salad
Steamed vegetables with picante sauce
Baked apple
Any dessert recipe found in Part III
Everyday Bran Muffins
Dr. Jay's Blueberry Oat Bran Muffins
Frozen fruit (banana, strawberries, or pineapple)

Frozen fruit sorbet (blend frozen fruit in food processor or blender)
Fruit Smoothie
Steamed artichoke
Steamed corn on the cob
Baked potato
Home-made tortilla chips (corn tortillas baked in 400°F oven)

BEVERAGES

1. There's no need to drink large amounts of water or other liquid on the L.A. Diet Program. The wide variety of fruits, vegetables, soups, and such provide plenty of water. In addition, excessive protein, alcohol, and caffeine, which are not found on the L.A. Diet Program, cause water loss. The rule with liquids is drink according to your natural thirst. *Note*: Drink lots of water before, during, and after vigorous exercise if it's hot or if you are perspiring heavily.
2. Avoid caffeine-containing beverages such as coffee, tea, diet colas, and other soft drinks. Caffeine is a stimulant and may cause nervousness, headaches, feelings of anxiety, sleepless nights, and even panic attacks.
3. Roasted grain beverages such as Caffix, Bamboo, Postum, and Roastaroma have a coffeelike flavor but contain no caffeine. Hot water with lemon is also refreshing and satisfying. Good cold beverage choices include low-sodium carbonated mineral water flavored with a touch of fruit juice, low-sodium V-8 Juice, tomato juice (without salt), mild herb tea (no caffeine) with ice.

MENU PLANS

Each of the following menu plans provides approximately 1,200 calories and includes the recommended servings from the five food groups. The menus are designed to assist you in getting started with your food plan (italicized recipes can be found in Part III). Feel free to create new menus and add or substitute foods, depending on your weight loss goal and your taste. For example, those wanting to lose weight should emphasize foods with low caloric density such as soups, salads, and vegetables. Those wanting to maintain weight should emphasize foods slightly high in caloric density, such as breads, grains, and starchy vegetables. Keep your meal plans simple, practical, and tasty. Experiment with the many delicious and easy-to-prepare recipes in Part III.

MENU 1

Breakfast

½ cup hot cooked oatmeal
½ medium banana (sliced)
1 cup skim milk
Dash cinnamon
Herb tea

Snack

1 bowl raw vegetables
1 medium peach

Lunch

1 bowl hot vegetable soup
Large salad with no-oil dressing
1 slice whole wheat bread or roll
1 cup steamed broccoli spears
½ cup fresh strawberries

Snack

2 cups popcorn (no oil or salt)
Mineral water with fruit juice flavoring

Dinner

1 large salad
1 medium baked potato
3 ounces steamed fish
1 cup steamed carrots and green beans

Snack

1 medium apple, chopped and added to 6 ounces nonfat plain yogurt

MENU 2

Breakfast

1 serving Sunrise Frittata
1 slice whole wheat toast
½ grapefruit, sectioned
¼ cup Grazing Cream Cheese
Herbal tea or grain beverage

Snack

Steamed artichoke with lemon
Raw vegetables

Lunch

1 bowl hot Chicken and Chili Soup
1 slice hot Corn Bread
Large salad with sliced tomatoes
1 cup steamed asparagus spears

Snack

6 ounces nonfat plain yogurt with ½ cup fresh pineapple and dash of cinnamon

Dinner

½ cup whole wheat noodles
1 cup Spaghetti Sauce
Large salad

Snack

1 slice Blueberry Cheesecake with Fruit Topping
Herb tea

MENU 3

Breakfast

1 slice French Toast
½ medium banana (sliced over toast)
2 tablespoons Fruit Topping
1 cup skim milk

Snack

1 apple, sliced
Raw vegetables

Lunch

1 bowl Quick Corn Chowder
1 warmed pita bread stuffed with vegetables
1 cup steamed Chinese pea pods and red bell pepper
1 medium peach, sliced

Snack

½ water bagel, toasted, with mustard
Tomato and onion slices

Dinner

1 serving Baked Halibut and Peppers
½ cup brown and wild rice
1 cup sliced cucumbers, tomatoes, and carrots
½ cup sliced kiwifruit

Snack

½ cup frozen banana
½ cup plain nonfat yogurt

MENU 4

Breakfast
½ cup hot cooked whole grain cereal
2 tablespoons raisins
1 cup skim milk

Snack

1 medium orange
Raw vegetables

Lunch

1 bowl Festive Soup
1 slice whole wheat bread
1 cup steamed zucchini and carrots
Large salad

Snack

6 ounces plain nonfat yogurt
½ cup blueberries

Dinner

1 serving Clams Linguini
1 cup steamed asparagus
Tossed green salad

Snack
1 slice No-Bake Strawberry Pie
½ cup Blueberry-Pineapple Topping

MENU 5

Breakfast

1 Everyday Bran Muffin
¼ melon
¼ cup Grazing Cream Cheese
Hot grain beverage

Snack

Hot vegetable soup
2–3 whole grain crackers

Lunch

Sandwich:
  2 slices whole wheat bread
  1 cup raw vegetables
  2 ounces tuna (water-packed)
12 green grapes

Snack

1 cup steamed vegetables with salsa to flavor

Dinner

1 slice Quick and Easy Pizza
Large salad with assorted vegetables

Snack

1 baked apple

MENU 6

Breakfast

1–2 Oatmeal Pancakes
¼ cup Fruit Topping
1 cup skim milk

Snack

Raw vegetables
1 medium orange

Lunch

Crepes *filled with Oriental vegetables*
1 bowl hot soup
½ cup assorted fresh fruit

Snack

½ English muffin with no-sugar fruit spread
Raw vegetables

Dinner

½ cup brown rice
1 serving Chicken Curry *with condiments: diced green and red bell pepper, water chestnuts, raisins*
Large green salad with slices of tomato
Fresh apple slices

Snack

6 ounces yogurt with 1 tablespoon apple juice concentrate

MENU 7

Breakfast

½ *cup* Sunny Morning Potatoes
Sliced tomatoes
1 cup skim milk
1 cup fresh fruit

Snack

Raw vegetables
Mineral water

Lunch

1 bowl Lentil Soup
Large salad
1 whole wheat roll, warmed
1 cup steamed green beans and carrots

Snack

6 ounces plain nonfat yogurt
½ *banana*

Dinner

1 serving Seafood Creole
½ *cup cooked barley*
Tossed green salad
1 cup steamed yellow squash

Snack

½ *cup frozen fruit*

13

EATING AWAY FROM HOME

"Join me for a bite of lunch." "Can you make it to my dinner party?" "I'm traveling back east for business." "Let's get together for cocktails." Dining out, entertaining, socializing, and traveling are a few of the special situations that play a role in our daily schedule and require us to eat away from home.

With the growing number of people eating out, whether for pleasure or business, there is a real concern about the food selections we're making. As a rule, foods that are typically high in fat, cholesterol, sugar, salt, and calories are associated with celebration, festivity, and socializing. This can present a host of new eating problems for the grazing diner. Restaurants offer many different tempting foods, often in large quantities and in an atmosphere of relaxation and unlimited eating. In the office, it's not uncommon to socialize with co-workers, surrounded by food, or to be involved in business conducted over a meal. In social situations such as banquets, buffets, parties, or a dinner at a friend's home, you are generally expected if not forced to overindulge. Also, holidays, vacations, and travel experiences are especially conducive to eating excessive quantities of food and drink. We overemphasize food, making it our main focus, and ignore the impact on and consequences to our health.

Fortunately, the times are changing. More people are choosing to eat lighter and healthier foods. In addition, hundreds of restaurants across the country—from the fast-food establishments to the major hotel chain operations—are making a concerted effort to include on their menus dishes that are lower in fat and calories. Food selections are expanding to include salad bars, whole grains, entrees without oils and butters, and fresh fruit combinations for desserts. Restaurateurs are also willing to accommodate the health-seeking patron by preparing meals as requested, eliminating ingredients or leaving accompaniments such as sauces and dressings on the side. Major travel operations such as airlines and cruise ship carriers are offering special meal selections such as "low-cholesterol" and "strict vegetarian" alternatives to meet the special dietary needs of their customers. In short, healthy eating is in vogue. The focus of businesses involved in meal preparation is on food that not only tastes good but is good for you.

Although eating out on the L.A. Diet Program is becoming easier, it's important to be armed with the insight and knowledge to handle any event that requires you to eat away from your own kitchen. Whether you are dining in a new restaurant or traveling abroad for business, the following tips and techniques will help you stick to the guidelines of the L.A. Diet Program. Use your imagination and open yourself up to new opportunities while eating away from home. Remember, this can be a fun challenge. You'll come out a winner without compromising your health or social life.

PLAN AHEAD

Make a commitment to plan your eating strategy in advance. Call ahead to a restaurant to inquire about its ability to honor special dietary requests, notify friends of your new eating program, and take food such as fruit or bread with you when traveling to ease potentially uncomfortable or difficult situations. This is especially important as you make the transition to your new eating program. Initially, most people find it easier to eat at home until they're better able to handle the challenges of eating out. However, once you're comfortable with the techniques of healthy dining, eating away from home becomes an enjoyable experience.

HAVE AN ALTERNATE GAME PLAN

It's wise to establish a second plan of action in any event involved with meals or food away from home. This technique is especially important when traveling. Carrying some food items with you such as fruit, bread, bagels, cut-up vegetables, or homemade sandwiches provides you with another option in case you're unable to select appropriate foods. Airports are a good example of the importance of having a second game plan. It's very common for planes to be delayed or, if requesting a special meal, to have your meal not show up. Therefore, a piece of fruit or slice of bread can get you through those tough times.

AVOID GOING OUT ON AN EMPTY STOMACH

This may appear to be an unusual suggestion for someone who is planning to attend a function involved with food. However, if you're very hungry when you're eating away from home, chances are you'll be tempted to make poor food choices. In addition, don't skip a meal in order to save up your calories for the next one. Rather, take the edge off your appetite by nibbling on salad, popcorn, or other grazing foods. Remember, on the L.A. Diet Program it's important to snack and eat smaller, more frequent meals throughout the day. You should never allow yourself to get very hungry before starting to eat.

MAKE THE BEST POSSIBLE CHOICES
WHENEVER POSSIBLE

Learn to prioritize your food choices when dining out. Foods high in fat are the major items to avoid, whereas foods containing refined ingredients or small amounts of sugar are certainly not as deleterious to your program. Compromise sensibly, but don't allow eating away from home to give you an excuse to give up your grazing guidelines.

HAVE A POSITIVE ATTITUDE

One of the most important tools for making your eating experience both
enjoyable and successful is taking on a positive attitude. Remember, you
are taking the responsibility of eating away from home. Therefore, your
attitude becomes your responsibility as well. Maintaining a good attitude not only helps you enjoy the L.A. Diet Program a great deal more
but it also helps encourage a positive response from those with whom
you interact. Waiters and waitresses are much more willing to oblige
your special requests. Also, friends and family are more cooperative in
helping you adapt to your new eating program. In short, a positive spirit
about your new way of eating helps you enjoy the challenges as you grow
in your knowledge of and experience with eating away from home.

Ultimately, these five major guidelines should assist you in any special
situation in which you'll be eating away from home. Just how many of
those special occasions you encounter may or may not be in your control. Often, there will be annual or seasonal events such as holidays,
anniversaries, and birthdays. Other times, where you go may not be of
your choosing, such as when you must travel for business. Let's take a
look at some common eating-away-from-home situations.

RESTAURANT DINING

Eating out in restaurants has become a national pastime. A warm and
elegant ambiance, the pleasure of good friends, and the enjoyment of a
cooked meal without having to lift a finger are but a few of the reasons
for the growing popularity of dining out. In addition, our fast-paced
lifestyles and the movement toward both women and men in the working world contribute to dining out. Americans eat out on the average of
four times each week. We spend over 35 percent of our food dollars in
restaurants. With the growing number of individuals eating in restaurants, there is a real concern about the food choices people are making.
Until now, most restaurants focused on food that simply tasted good
without concern over the consequences to our health.

Fortunately for the grazing patron, many more options are now available to help you enjoy both the food and the pleasure of eating meals

outside the home. From fine dining, white-tablecloth operations to small-town diners and fast-food establishments, health-conscious choices are becoming available. On almost every menu, you'll find items such as salads, soups, light appetizers, or lean entrees. In addition, "spa dining" has penetrated many of the major hotel and restaurant establishments. This term is used to suggest lower-calorie menu options. To guide you in selecting the best possible food and menu choices, experiment with the following suggestions.

Choosing a Restaurant

Be as selective as possible when deciding where to dine out. Choose restaurants that cater to the health-conscious diner whenever possible. Many restaurants are including fresh vegetables, salads, and salad bars. Lower-fat alternatives to red meat such as chicken and fish are also provided. Avoid the "all-you-can-eat" restaurants that have feasts designed for the "gorgers." Often the food lacks quality taste and is only plentiful in quantity. Also, think twice before choosing a traditional restaurant, noted for its cream- and sauce-based dishes.

The most reliable restaurant choices for the health-seeking diner include seafood restaurants, salad bar establishments, and fine hotel and restaurant chains. Several types of ethnic restaurants, such as Japanese, Chinese, Italian, and Mexican, also present a variety of meal options. In addition, many restaurants across the nation are serving foods approved by the American Heart Association. The foods must meet the Association's specific guidelines for fat and cholesterol. Although these guidelines are not in complete sync with the L.A. Diet Program (fat, cholesterol, and salt levels are higher), there is the potential for ordering the dishes to your liking.

Selecting Your Food

What to eat for breakfast, lunch, and dinner while dining out may seem a bit ambiguous when you don't know in advance what a restaurant will offer. However, there are some general guidelines that should provide assistance in making these decisions.

BREAKFAST

Hot cereals are your best choice when dining out for breakfast. The warmth of the cereal has a double bonus of filling you up nutritionally while satisfying your appetite and hunger. Remember, you're likely to eat less when you fill up on hot foods, especially high-carbohydrate foods. Oatmeal is a popular choice served in most any restaurant, whether it be a standard coffeehouse or a fine hotel. Cream of Wheat is another option. Although this is not a whole grain cereal, it still can be an appropriate choice because it contains no cholesterol or added fat, sugar, or salt. Be sure to order your cereal cooked in water, not cream or milk, and to request that no salt or sugar be added. Some restaurants may present the option of having fruit such as sliced bananas, raisins, or blueberries cooked into your cereal, which is a nice treat. Ordering a bowl of fresh fruit on the side is also a refreshing addition to your breakfast meal.

Other breakfast choices include whole grain English muffins, water bagels, or pumpernickel, rye, or whole wheat bread. Have these toasted dry without butter. Instead, use a small amount of jam or fruit preserve to provide a sweet flavor or use mustard or salsa for a nice savory taste. You can take the bread choices a step further and ask for sliced tomatoes, lettuce, and onions and create an excellent sandwich. This is especially good on a bagel.

Egg-based dishes are highly visible on the breakfast menu, from three-egg omelets to scrambled eggs and bacon. For obvious reasons (300 milligrams of cholesterol per egg yolk!), it makes sense to avoid these traditional dishes. However, you might consider requesting an egg-white omelet. Ask if the chef can sauté a variety of vegetables such as onions, peppers, tomatoes, mushrooms, or sprouts in a small amount of liquid (as opposed to oil) and combine them with just the egg white, no yolks. Surprisingly, more restaurants nationwide are accommodating this request. Hotel restaurants are also providing the option of a low-cholesterol omelet by using Egg Beaters in place of the eggs. This is a nice healthy option to consider. However, whenever ordering a food item off the grill, be sure to specify that it be cooked with as little oil or butter as possible. Flavor your egg-white dishes with salsa or picante sauce, which adds a nice spicy bite.

Pancakes, waffles, and French toast are usually best avoided. Generally, they're prepared from premade batters that include eggs, whole milk, oil, or butter. The more health-conscious restaurant may cook to order or use less of these ingredients, so whether these are possible choices will depend on the restaurant. Again, ask for the cooking to be done as dry as possible, and request no butter to be added. Fresh fruit makes for an excellent topping, or a small amount of syrup can be spread lightly over the pancakes without doing much harm.

Other breakfast choices could include cold cereal such as Shredded Wheat or Grapenuts if the restaurant provides these options. If not, order a low-sugar, high-fiber cereal such as All Bran or 40% Bran. Use skim milk or fruit juice instead of low-fat or whole milk, or bring your own powdered nonfat milk powder and dilute with water.

Be wary of bran muffins, which seem to have swept across the nation as a trendy delicacy. A seemingly harmless muffin can have anywhere between 200 and 400 calories per serving if made with eggs, oil, and sugar. If nothing else seems appropriate, this could be a relatively good choice. However, be cautious—ask how the bran muffins are prepared and use your own discretion.

LUNCH AND DINNER

Choose a restaurant that will provide a number of choices when eating lunch or dinner away from home. You may wish to call ahead to a new restaurant and ask what's on the menu. Also, find out if the establishment will honor special dietary requests. Remember, too, avoid dining out when you are famished. Nibble on some crackers, popcorn, veggies, or fruit. However, if the luncheon or dinner event is a special occasion and you wish to enjoy more than a salad, then do not eat too much before going out. This kind of planning ahead is important in helping you gain control over your eating habits. Too many times people gorge on special-occasion meals and feel the consequences the next day.

Your best choices for lunch include salads, vegetable plates, hot bread without butter, sandwiches, and light entrees that may include fish. When ordering a salad, be sure to request that the dressing be kept to the side. Most people don't realize the dietary disaster they cause by using salad dressing. A large salad comprised of raw vegetables such as carrots, lettuce, cucumbers, sprouts, beets, broccoli, cauliflower, spinach, and other salad options can amount to a mere 100 calories. However, when you add $\frac{1}{4}$–$\frac{1}{2}$ cup of dressing, which is a typical amount for most people, you're adding between 350 and 700 calories! One tablespoon of dressing has 80–100 calories. For the same number of calories, you could have a baked potato, steamed broccoli, and a salad.

Be calorie wise, especially with fats. Remember, fat makes you fat by increasing your set point for body fat. Instead of salad dressing, you're much better off using fresh lemon, vinegar, Tabasco sauce, salsa, or a dash of soy sauce over your salad. Or, you may want to eat it plain. Learning to taste the refreshing flavors of vegetables can be a great sensory experience for your palate.

Avoid all preprepared salads that are made with oils, mayonnaise, cold cuts, cheeses, eggs, and marinated vegetables. Avocado, nuts, seeds, and olives are also popular salad fixings that are discouraged because of their high fat content.

Another lunch option includes a variety of sandwiches. Order your sandwich on either grain bread or a bagel. Hold the mayonnaise. Ask for mustard only. Add lettuce, tomato, sprouts, or any other vegetable. You may want to ask for a thin layer of white turkey meat for your sandwich.

A hot bowl of a clear or tomato-based soup makes for a satisfying addition to your lunch. Be aware that most restaurant soups tend to be high in salt. Therefore, choose soup only occasionally when low-sodium options are available. Good soup choices include vegetable, red-based Manhattan clam chowder, split pea, minestrone, and lentil.

Dinner choices are similar to the luncheon ideas. However, you may wish to expand and look at other menu offerings. Be sure to scan the entire menu. Consider the appetizers, soups, salads, and à la carte options in addition to the entrees. Unless you're going to share dinner, you're better off ordering smaller portions to avoid eating more than you need. Fish and other animal-based foods generally come in smaller portions when found in the appetizer section. For example, an order of steamed oysters, mussels, or clams can make a nice complement to a salad, bowl of soup, and hot bread. Other dinner options include pasta or rice and steamed vegetables served with a meatless marinara sauce. Include a salad and some fresh berries for dessert for a satisfying meal.

Avoid deep-fried chicken or fish. When ordering poultry, avoid duck and goose. They contain all dark meat and are very high in fat. Chicken and Cornish game hens are your best bet. Always remove the skin before eating.

Fish is generally the best option when ordering animal protein. It is usually lower in fat, cholesterol, and calories than poultry or meat. Any cold water, flat white fish or mollusk is an excellent choice. Some suggestions include flounder, sole, halibut, salmon, mackerel, red snapper, bass, swordfish, scallops, mussels, oysters, clams, and squid. Lobster, crab, and shrimp are higher in cholesterol and should be eaten less often and in smaller portions. Order fish or chicken poached in wine, steamed, baked, broiled, or grilled without butter. Watch serving sizes. You may wish to split the order or take half home in a doggy bag to avoid eating more protein, fat, and cholesterol than you need.

Don't forget about the infamous baked potato, which can be a meal in itself. Although considered a calorically dense food, the potato's nutritional benefits make the calories count. Try salsa, soy sauce, lemon, or Tabasco over your potato to add flavor. A plain baked potato is also a nice addition to a fresh salad or bowl of soup.

Ethnic Restaurants

Ethnic restaurants provide many options for the grazing diner. The following is a summary of menu suggestions and guidelines for the various types of restaurants generally found. Keep a list of some of your favorite dining establishments and refer to this list when you wish to dine out or suggest a restaurant to another health-conscious diner.

CHINESE

Choose steamed or lightly stir-fried entrees. Ask if your entree can be stir-fried with defatted chicken stock or water as opposed to oil. Request that no salt or MSG be added to your food. Avoid fried foods such as fried rice and noodles, and skip the sweet and sour dishes. Good choices include steamed vegetables, rice or translucent noodles and diced white chicken meat, fish, or tofu (soybean curd). Several good choices in a Chinese restaurant include moo goo gai pan (chicken, vegetables, and rice), chicken or vegetable chop suey (chicken, vegetables, and translucent noodles), Buddha's delight (a good vegetarian dish prepared with tofu—request it steamed), and any clear-based soups prepared with vegetables, tofu, or rice. Avoid Chinese tea as it contains caffeine—try hot water with lemon or any herbal tea without caffeine.

ITALIAN

Select pastas prepared without eggs to avoid additional fat and cholesterol in your meal. You may need to ask how the pasta is made, to determine the presence of egg yolks. To reduce the caloric density of your meals, have a light meatless marinara, tomato, Neapolitan, or red clam sauce. Avoid heavy cream, olive oil, and cheese-based dishes. Fresh salads without the dressing, hot Italian bread (without butter), pasta and vegetables, minestrone soup, and seafood dishes are good choices in an Italian restaurant. Linguini with red clam sauce or other red-based fish sauces are good choices. Another excellent and enjoyable option to choose is pizza. Order it with extra vegetables such as onions, peppers, mushrooms, zucchini, or chopped green chilies over a meatless marinara sauce, garnish with fresh garlic, and hold the cheese. This is a surprisingly delicious entree that can be served with a fresh salad or bowl of soup for a nice satisfying meal. Fresh steamed vegetables such as artichoke, zucchini, and eggplant may be found on the menu. Avoid deep-fried and batter-coated dishes, olives, veal, and other meats such as sausage.

MEXICAN

Food choices in a Mexican restaurant can be worked into the L.A. Diet Program: corn tortillas, boiled beans, and vegetables such as lettuce, tomato, onions, corn, and potatoes. Fresh red or green chili salsa is an excellent accompaniment to meals. A warning to the grazing diner trying to lose weight is that the caloric density of Mexican or Southwestern foods is high. Many of the starch-based foods are fine to incorporate into your new eating program, however, exercise portion control. Emphasize lighter, less calorically dense foods such as the vegetables.

Tortilla chips are plentiful in the Mexican restaurant but are generally fried. Instead, ask for the chips to be baked or order a plate of steamed corn tortillas. Frijoles, which are beans, are a good choice, but ask that they be prepared in water or broth instead of being refried in lard. Calling ahead to the restaurant earlier in the day (preferably in the morning) and requesting an order of beans to be set aside before refrying is one option to try.

To reduce the caloric density of your meal, choose Mexican dishes that emphasize larger portions of vegetables. For example, tostadas can be made with small amounts of chicken or beans and larger amounts of shredded lettuce, tomatoes, chilies, bell peppers, and salsa. Be sure to avoid sour cream, avocado or guacamole, cheese, and deep-fried foods. Ask that these items be left off your plate. Instead, ask for side orders of steamed tortillas, beans, vegetables, and rice. Often chicken or bean fajitas are included on the menu. Several side dishes can be arranged, and you can simply build your meal with any of the accompaniments. Other selections such as gazpacho, seafood dishes such as red snapper Veracruz and ceviche (marinated fish), and chicken or bean enchiladas are all good menu options.

FRENCH

Fortunately, many French chefs are becoming familiar with light and healthy methods for preparing French cuisine. Gourmet French restaurants throughout the country are reforming their style of cooking from the traditional techniques. However, always ask that the sauces be left to the side. Opt for chicken, fish, or other seafood dishes and request that they be prepared by a method such as poaching, steaming, baking, or broiling without butter. Avoid *au gratin* dishes, cream-based dishes, rich sauces such as béarnaise, béchamel, and hollandaise.

Steamed vegetables, salads, or vegetable casseroles may be on the menu. Look for the term *spa cuisine* for light and lower-fat options. Avoid crepes, quiches, and other egg-based dishes. French bread is refined but does not contain butter or oil. Have a slice with dinner if you choose. Fresh fruit such as melon or berries makes for a nice refreshing dessert.

JAPANESE

Similar to Chinese cuisine, Japanese food can be appropriate for the grazing diner when chosen with discretion. Foods are generally prepared light and without many rich sauces or dressings. The most important concern, however, is the high salt content of the food. Soy sauce, miso, pickled vegetables, and salted fish are all part of the Japanese menu and represent high-sodium foods. Avoid these foods whenever possible and opt for fresh foods without seasoning. Several menu options to consider include steamed vegetables, rice, salads with the dressing on the side, fish, and noodles. The popular choices in a Japanese restaurant include sashimi (raw fish) and sushi (raw fish with rice).

Soups can be a nice choice to have with your meal. Watch out for salted soups made with miso or kelp (seaweed). Request a clear-based broth soup with vegetables or other acceptable ingredients. Condiments to use in the Japanese restaurant include fresh ginger, hot mustard, vinegars, and small amounts of soy sauce. Request that no MSG, sugar, or salt be added to your food.

SEAFOOD RESTAURANTS

Restaurants specializing in seafood dishes are a good and safe choice for the grazing diner. Most all seafood can be enjoyed on the L.A. Diet Program, provided the method of preparation is appropriate. Good fish choices include halibut, sea bass, swordfish, red snapper, salmon, flounder, scallops, clams, oysters, and other mollusks. Have the fish broiled, steamed, grilled, or baked with wine or lemon juice. Avoid butter, bread, or batter coating and deep-fried seafood.

A new trend that is hitting many new American cuisine restaurants is the Cajun or "blackened" fish. Although the spices used in this process are acceptable, there is quite a bit of salt added and in some cases, oil is used. In addition, "blackening" is a method of exposing the fish to excessive charring, which may pose a health concern with respect to its carcinogenic potential. This menu choice would certainly be fine if chosen on an occasional basis. If possible, ask for it to be prepared lightly and without the salt. The spices add a nice zesty flavor and have a favorable effect on your metabolic rate.

Be sure to portion-control your fish entrees. Order fish from the appetizer section of the menu or eat half of a regular entree portion. This helps you reduce your dietary intake of protein, fat, and cholesterol. Fill the rest of your plate instead with salad, a baked potato or rice, and a red-based fish soup such as Manhattan clam chowder.

STEAKHOUSES

Most steakhouses have a very complete salad bar with a variety of fresh raw vegetables. You may wish to bring your own salad dressing or use lemon, vinegar, or salsa. Avoid any of the already prepared salads. Baked potatoes are also a common staple in steakhouses, and they make a nice complement to a large salad. Be sure to order your potato without butter or sour cream. Instead, stuff your potato with salad or use some appropriate condiments such as Tabasco, mustard, or small amounts of steak sauce for flavor. Avoid fried foods such as french fries or hash brown potatoes. Meat choices are typically high-fat (especially saturated fat, which increases cholesterol levels), high-calorie menu items, which should be avoided.

FAST-FOOD RESTAURANTS

Fortunately, the fast-food restaurant chains across the country are responding to the consumer demand for healthier and lighter foods. Typically, a fast-food restaurant is a haven for high-salt, high-fat, high-cholesterol, and high-calorie menu options. One double beef Whopper with cheese has 980 calories! And that doesn't include the french fries and beverage. It's no wonder Americans are getting fatter. Today, however, you can dine in a fast-food restaurant without destroying your new eating program. Opt for the chains that offer salad bars. You can stock up on nutrient-rich vegetables such as dark green lettuce, tomatoes, sprouts, beets, cucumbers, and a variety of fresh fruits. In addition, whole wheat pita bread, baked potatoes, and steamed corn on the cob are available at some restaurants. It's best to stay away from any of the prepared sandwiches that contain meat, deep-fried fish, or chicken. Some chicken-based chains may offer broiled chicken prepared on a roaster, which would be an acceptable choice. Beverages generally contain sugar or artificial sweeteners. You may be able to spot a club soda or mineral water on the menu. Juices, although more concentrated in calories, can be combined with the mineral water to make a refreshing beverage.

Additional Tips

Remember to keep an open mind when you dine out at any restaurant. The following are tips worth noting:
  1. Go easy on the alcohol. Try to limit yourself to one drink by ordering a nonalcoholic beverage (tomato juice, carbonated mineral water, or fruit juice) as a predinner drink. If you choose to have a drink, select one that is low in alcohol content such as a wine spritzer or a light beer.

Alcohol has a great ability to decrease your resistance to tempting foods. Also, it's high in calories with no appreciable nutrient value. (More about this subject in the discussion of cocktail parties.)

2. Be specific when ordering your food and communicate clearly the nature of your order. Don't assume the waiter or waitress will know to leave the cheese off your steamed vegetables even though you requested "no butter." Ask plenty of questions about how the food is prepared. Remember, this is your meal and you are paying for it to be prepared and presented in the manner that you desire.

3. Don't be afraid to send back a dish if it's not prepared appropriately. If you asked for your food to be made a specific way and you find that it comes covered in a rich sauce or butter, be sure to speak up and request that it be prepared again. You need not make a scene in sending back your food. Be kind and courteous but firm.

4. Avoid feeling obligated to eat everything on your plate. There's no need to stuff yourself with food because you feel you've paid for it. This is the gorging style of most Americans. Taking a doggy bag home with left-over portions is a great way to solve this problem. In addition, you have a meal for lunch the next day, which saves time in the kitchen. Remember, on the L.A. Diet Program it's important to avoid eating too much food at one time. Having small, more frequent meals is the preferred way to feed the body.

COCKTAIL PARTIES, BANQUETS, BUFFETS, AND ENTERTAINING

Most likely in the near future you will attend a function at someone else's request. It may be a holiday cocktail party, office get-together, banquet, buffet, or dinner at someone's home. In some instances, you may be the one giving the gala event. Whatever the case may be, you can still avoid compromising your health, food choices, or desired weight loss goal.

The following are suggestions for making these special-occasion events enjoyable experiences.

Cocktail Parties and Other Social Events

At cocktail events, avoid drinking to your heart's content. Limit alcohol consumption for the obvious health reasons and because of its high caloric density. If you choose to drink, make your first drink a nonalcoholic beverage. This will slow your pace, since the first drink at a cocktail party is usually consumed at a faster rate than subsequent drinks. The more alcohol you consume, the more it will affect you and the more likely you are to give in to tempting, high-calorie foods.

Nonalcoholic beverages include mineral water with a splash of fruit juice, tonic water with a twist of lime, or club soda by itself. Tomato juice, fruit juice, or carbonated water such as club soda with cranberry or other fruit juice can be a refreshing alternative to alcoholic beverages. However, if you do plan to have a cocktail or dinner drink, choose one that is lower in alcohol content. For example, fruit- or vegetable-based drinks provide nutrients and help to dilute the alcohol absorption. Wine spritzers (dry white wine and club soda) are another lighter drink. Dry wine, light beer, or an occasional glass of champagne can also be enjoyed without causing too much harm.

Ignore the high-fat, high-calorie chips, dips, canapes, and nuts. No one can eat just one of these snacks. They're easy to overconsume and add more salt and fat to your diet. Rather, opt for the relish tray and nibble on raw vegetables, fruits, and dry crisp crackers. It's best to stand far from the hors d'oeuvres table and focus your attention on the pleasure and conversation of the guests. The fact that the food and drinks are present does not mean you need to indulge. Grazing on acceptable light snacks before attending these kinds of functions is an asset in disguise. Such a snack will prevent you from being too hungry, which could lead to a dietary disaster.

Banquets and Buffets

Whenever it is possible, try to find out what will be served when planning to attend a buffet or banquet. This can help you plan your strategy accordingly. If the menu is not appropriate, you can have your dinner at home and eat very little at the event. A buffet or banquet-style meal allows for freedom in food selection and control over portion sizes. It's up to you to decide how much or what kind of food to eat. It's possible in these situations to be quite moderate in your food choices and portion sizes.

Choose salad whenever possible, but avoid the dressing. If you plan to eat the entree, make it as acceptable as possible. Scrape off sauces, trim off any visible fat, and remove breading or cheese. Look for boiled or baked potatoes, steamed vegetables, and fresh fruit. Remember to do the best you can. It may not always be possible to get the "perfect" grazing meal. By making the best choices whenever possible, you will be doing much more for your health than not. Also, keep in mind what foods are most important to avoid. Fat- and cholesterol-containing foods will do much more harm than a small amount of cocktail sauce that may contain sugar.

Entertaining with Friends

Being honest and open about your dietary quest is probably the best way to deal with entertaining or dining at a friend's home. This can ease a potentially uncomfortable situation. Enlist the understanding and support of the host or hostess by informing him or her that you are on a special eating program. You never know when friends or other acquaintances may be following a similar diet. Today it's unlikely that you'll find yourself alone in trying to watch the fat, calories, and cholesterol in your food. In advance, ask if sauces, dressings, or butter can be left off your portion of food or offer to bring a dish to share at the social gathering. This way you're guaranteed something acceptable to eat.

Make a special effort to praise your host or hostess for the social event in and of itself and don't apologize for not overindulging in food or wine. When friends understand that you are caring for your health, they will be less likely to be offended when you don't eat any of their creative culinary dishes. Often, too, you may wish to have one or two bites of a delicacy. This is certainly not an unhealthy compromise. In fact, it may take some of the inquisitive nature away from your palate.

When entertaining in your own home, life on the L.A. Diet Program doesn't necessarily get easier. How do you accommodate everyone's taste buds and not forfeit your new eating program? Simply, experiment with some of the recipes from Chapter 15 and serve some delicious, creative, and exciting dishes. This can be a rewarding challenge. At first, you may want to practice some recipes on your family or close friends. This way you have a better idea of how your new cuisine will be received.

Don't force food and drink on your company. Allow them to experiment at their own pace. You may wish to offer two kinds of cuisine—one that is prepared following the guidelines of the L.A. Diet Program and one that is a modified version—when entertaining. In this way your friends can choose what they want to eat, and you can have a meal to enjoy as well. This is a helpful party alternative to consider around the holiday season when most people are inclined toward overeating and indulging in food and drink.

TRAVELING

It is easier today for the grazing traveler to eat lightly while dining away from home. A number of hotels now cater to you by offering menu selections for special diets. The guidelines outlined in the restaurant section of this chapter apply just as well to dining away from home.

Traveling for business or pleasure can exacerbate unpleasant physical conditions such as fatigue, dehydration, lack of sleep, and irregular eating habits. To combat these physical ailments, you need to plan ahead.

If traveling by plane, request a special meal in advance. Most airlines offer menu alternatives such as low-cholesterol, low-fat, strict vegetarian, diabetic, low-sodium, and low-calorie plates in addition to other options. Each airline carrier will differ in its food choices, and you may not always get what you thought you had ordered. Some of the better choices include the strict vegetarian, fruit plate, and low-cholesterol options. You may wish to ask in advance what's offered on each of the menus. Also, it's important to take a few food items with you while you travel. You never know when your plane may be delayed or when the special meal won't make it to your seat. Snacking on a bagel, piece of fruit, or vegetables can help get you to your destination.

Avoid drinking alcoholic beverages and caffeine-containing drinks such as coffee, tea, or cola. Such beverages actually accentuate the loss of body fluids that you already experience from the dry air found in planes. Sip carbonated water, seltzer or club soda, and small amounts of fruit juice. Because fruit juice contains potassium, it can alleviate the loss in body fluids.

When traveling by car, carry a cooler stocked with food such as nonfat yogurt, fruit, canned tuna, bagels, and breads. Include condiments such as mustard, salsa, and horseradish to use over vegetables or on sandwiches. When your food supply runs low, you can always restock at a grocery store in any town. This method of traveling can be a lot of fun. You'll feel more energetic by grazing throughout the day.

Traveling by boat on a major cruise line can also work into your new grazing lifestyle. Be sure to call at least two weeks in advance to request your special meal plan. Every cruise carrier operates differently, so check with your travel agent for information on special meal services. Also, plan to bring several food staples with you to make your meals more palatable, such as salad dressing, nonfat milk powder for your cereal, herbal seasonings, whole grain breads or crackers, and herbal tea bags.

The grazing guidelines are easiest to follow once you've gained knowledge, confidence, and experience in handling unusual or special situations. We've provided many tips and techniques for best handling these events. Now it's up to you to go out there and take on the challenge of eating away from home. Remember, make the journey to healthy eating fun and enjoyable. Enjoy the process of learning and use your creative imagination to select the best possible food choices for your grazing program!

III

RECIPES FOR GRAZING YOUR WAY TO HEALTH

by Diane M. Grabowski, M.N.S., R.D.

Healthy food need not be bland, or deprive the palate of flavor and taste. Rather, grazing recipes can open the door to discovering multitudes of delicious and satisfying meals. This part of the book explores a wide horizon of healthy, light, and elegant recipes representing the new grazing cuisine. We'll discuss the principles of low-fat, low-cholesterol, and low-sodium cooking, providing tips and helpful hints for making the transition to your L.A. Diet Program easier. With a little imagination and creativity you can master healthful cooking without sacrificing pleasure, your waistline, and, most importantly, your health.

The recipes are divided into seven chapters: soups; salads and vegetables; sauces, dressings, and dips; light entrees; breads and grains; desserts and snacks; and beverages.

The recipes that follow are designed to provide you with a foundation to start your new eating plan. Many of the dishes are good family-style recipes. Others are elegant and tasteful enough to serve at parties or other social gatherings. Nutritional analysis* is provided at the end of

*Values based on data from Bowes and Church's *Food Values of Portions Commonly Used*, 14th edition, 1985. Total values may not equal 100 due to rounding of numbers and variation in conversion factors.

each recipe. The analysis includes the important items to be concerned with: cholesterol, fat, sodium, protein, carbohydrates, and calories. Use this information for a better understanding of the foods you are eating and the health value they contribute to your diet.

The following list is a guide to sensible substitutions to help you get started with your new grazing cuisine. Use these to adapt your old favorite recipes and to create new ones as you go.

SENSIBLE SUBSTITUTIONS

INSTEAD OF:	TRY:
whole eggs	egg white (2 per egg)
whole milk	skim milk or evaporated skim milk
cream cheese	*Grazing Cream Cheese*
sour cream	*Grazing Sour Cream*
luncheon meats	turkey or chicken breast, skinless, white meat
butter or margarine	defatted broth or other oilless liquid
white flour	whole wheat flour or whole wheat pastry flour
creamed cottage cheese	nonfat dry-curd cottage cheese or 1% cottage cheese (rinse with water to remove cream)
heavy cream	evaporated skim milk, nonfat milk powder (added to liquid skim milk)
mayonnaise	*Grazing Creamy Salad Dressing* or nonfat yogurt with added lemon juice, dry mustard, and herbs
oil for sautéing	defatted chicken broth, wine, or vegetable juice
oil for baking	mashed banana, blueberries, applesauce, or other fruit
sugar or honey	apple or pineapple juice concentrate, unsweetened, undiluted
ice cream	frozen fruit blended or mixed
salt	lemon juice, herb and spice blends without salt
soy sauce	low-sodium soy sauce (in small amounts)
hamburgers	lean flank or round steak, ground
candy	dried fruit (dates, raisins, apricots)
nuts and crackers	popcorn (no oil or salt), baked corn tortillas, rice crackers, or any acceptable cracker
cakes, pastries	grazing desserts such as cheesecakes, pies, and muffins
red meats, duck, ham, pork	fish and poultry (chicken and turkey breasts)

14
SOUPS:
WARM UP AND SLIM DOWN

What could be more satisfying than a hot bowl of soup for pleasing both palate and appetite? A steaming bowl of soup can do wonders—chasing away the chill on a cold crisp day while warming you up and slimming you down.

Soups are nutritionally satisfying and excellent for encouraging weight loss due to their ability to lower the fat "set point." Hot soup increases body temperature and affects the satiety factor of the brain, acting like a natural appetite suppressant that helps you to feel full and therefore eat less at a given meal.

Soup can be used as an appetizer, an entree, or a mid-morning or afternoon snack. The heartiness of the soup depends on the ingredients and the method by which you prepare them. The following tips can help you make the most of your soup recipes.

1. Reduce the calories in your soup by including a majority of lower-calorie vegetables such as carrots, onions, celery, and broccoli. Use a homemade defatted stock to increase flavor without salt, butter, or oils.
2. Increase calories in soup by including more of the starch-based foods such as pasta, beans, rice, or other grains.

3. Thicken soup by simmering slowly until the flavor is rich. Also, blending half of the soup and returning it to the pot to cook for a few minutes longer increases the body and texture. Blending potatoes and adding skim milk create creamier soups.

4. Leave the vegetable peels intact, such as with carrots, potatoes, turnips, and parsnips, for the best flavor and optimum nutrition when making both soup and stock.

5. Use plenty of herbs and spices to bring out the flavor of vegetables. (Refer to the herb list in Chapter 5.)

6. Most soups can be frozen. Simply cool to room temperature and store in airtight sealed containers. Be sure to label your containers with name and date. To serve, remove soup from freezer and reheat in a microwave or on the stove.

7. For time-saving steps, prepare your soup in a microwave oven or pressure cooker. Use a crockpot for the convenience in allowing soups to cook all day. Process vegetable ingredients such as onion, celery, and carrots in a food processor to save time in chopping.

We'll begin with our basic stock recipes, which are an invaluable flavor component in making soups. These stocks can be refrigerated for 48 hours and frozen for 6 months. Use stocks in place of oil for sautéing vegetables, herbs, chicken, fish, or in place of water to enrich the flavor of grains.

The process of defatting the stock is essential for reducing both fat and calories—the fundamental objective of the L.A. Diet Program. You'll be quite amazed by the amount of fat that can be rendered from one chicken. This alone will give you an appreciation for the importance of the defatting process.

BASIC CHICKEN STOCK

2–3 pounds chicken backs, necks, wings, and carcass
3 quarts water
1 large onion, peeled and halved
1 medium leek
1 large carrot
2 medium celery stalks, with leaves
1 clove garlic, peeled and crushed
½ cup chopped fresh parsley, with stems
1 teaspoon crushed dried red pepper
1 teaspoon dried thyme
1 bay leaf

1. Place chicken in an 8- to 10-quart pot. Add water to cover (about 3 quarts).

2. Cut onion, leek, carrot, and celery stalks into large chunks and add to pot. Add garlic, parsley, crushed red pepper, thyme, and bay leaf.

3. Bring chicken, vegetables, and seasonings to a boil. Allow to cook for 5 minutes, removing any residue or foam from the stock with a slotted spoon.

4. Reduce temperature to low. Leave partially covered and continue to cook for 2½ hours.

5. Set a large strainer or colander over a bowl. Pour and strain, separating liquid from chicken and vegetables. Place a layer of cheese-cloth or filter paper over liquid. Place in refrigerator overnight to allow the fat to rise.

6. Defat broth by removing cloth, chicken fat, and any residual fat particles.

7. Store defatted stock in freezer in various-sized containers and in ice cube trays (for bouillon cubes).

MAKES 3 QUARTS

calories per 1-cup serving	8	carbohydrate	0
cholesterol	0	sodium	0
fat	0	caloric density	10
protein	2 g (100%)		

- Time-saving tip: Use a pressure cooker and cook for approximately 40 minutes.

VARIATIONS

1. Cook a whole chicken overnight using a crock pot. Remove lean, white meat portions to be used in salads or entrees. Continue to cook the remainder of chicken with ingredients as mentioned above.

2. Turkey Stock: *Turkey broth may be made from the above recipe, using 2 pounds turkey carcass in place of chicken.*

3. Beef Stock: *Substitute 2 pounds beef for chicken in the above recipe to make beef stock.*

4. Fish Stock: *Substitute 2 pounds fish heads and bones to make a fish stock.*

5. Vegetable Stock: *To make a vegetable stock, double or triple vegetables listed in the Basic Chicken Stock recipe and eliminate the meat. Delete the defatting process. Don't discard the vegetables. Simply puree the combination for a richer stock or use as ingredients for soups or stews.*

COLORFUL VEGETABLE SOUP

This soup is light and nutritious. There is no one recipe for vegetable soup, so experiment with your own favorite vegetables and use seasonal vegetables as desired. For a thicker soup, cook longer or use more vegetables, pasta, potatoes, or grains.

3–4 cups Vegetable Stock or Basic Chicken Stock (see index for recipe)
1 carrot, diced
½ cup sliced onion
1–2 garlic cloves, minced
1–2 parsley sprigs
1 tablespoon dried basil
1 cup green beans, fresh or frozen
1 yellow squash, diced
1 zucchini, diced
1 cup diced broccoli
½ cup cooked or canned garbanzo beans (rinse, if using canned)
½ cup corn kernels, fresh or frozen

1. Combine stock, carrots, onion, garlic, parsley, and basil in large pot. Bring to boil and simmer 30 minutes.

2. Add green beans, yellow squash, zucchini, broccoli, and beans. Simmer 30 minutes. Add corn and cook 20 minutes longer. Season to taste.

VARIATIONS

1. Add 1 medium potato, diced, or 1 cup pasta along with the corn.
2. Add 1 cup barley or rice in step 1.

MAKES 3–4 SERVINGS

calories per 1-cup serving	122	carbohydrate	23 g (75%)
cholesterol	0	sodium	24 mg
fat	.7 g (5%)	caloric density	30
protein	6 g (20%)		

CARROT SOUP

½ large onion, cubed
¾ pound carrots, peeled and cubed
½ large potato, cubed
3 cups Basic Chicken Stock, defatted (see index for recipe)
¼ teaspoon ground cumin (optional)
1½ teaspoons rice vinegar
1 pinch freshly ground black pepper (optional)

1. *Separately, chop onion and carrot finely using a food processor and add to soup pot. Chop potato and add to pot.*

2. *Add chicken stock and cumin. Cover and heat to simmering for 5 minutes. Continue to cook, partially covered, until vegetables are tender and soup is thickened, about 30 minutes.*

3. *Puree half of soup mixture in a blender or food processor to thicken further or puree all if smooth texture is desired. Add vinegar and black pepper. Serve immediately or cool and refrigerate up to 36 hours. Reheat before serving.*

MAKES 4 SERVINGS

calories per serving	83	carbohydrate	17 g (82%)
cholesterol	0 mg	sodium	36 mg
fat	.2 g (2%)	caloric density	26
protein	2 g (10%)		

POTATO-BROCCOLI SOUP

2 medium potatoes, chopped
½ large bunch broccoli stalks, sliced
1 cup water
1 large leek, washed and sliced
¼ teaspoon dried thyme
⅛ teaspoon dried rosemary, crushed
⅛ teaspoon ground cumin
¼ teaspoon dried dill (optional)
1 cup skim milk
Freshly ground black pepper (optional)

1. *Steam potatoes and broccoli with 1 cup water until tender (about 10 minutes). Drain, reserving cooking liquid. Set aside.*

2. *Sauté the leek in a nonstick skillet using a small amount of vegetable spray or chicken stock, until soft. Add thyme, rosemary, cumin, and dill. Cook for 1 minute.*

3. *Puree potatoes, broccoli, leek mixture, milk, and ½ cup of the vegetable liquid (or chicken stock) in a blender or food processor until smooth. Add additional chicken stock if needed. Return to saucepan and garnish with black pepper.*

VARIATION

Serve hot or cold. Add more chicken stock to soup if a thinner consistency is desired.

MAKES 4 SERVINGS

calories per serving	88	carbohydrate	17 g (77%)
cholesterol	1 mg	sodium	44 mg
fat	.3 g (3%)	caloric density	53
protein	4 g (18%)		

TOMATO-RICE SOUP

½ cup long-grain brown rice, uncooked
1 cup chopped onion
2–3 celery ribs, including leaves or tops, chopped
2–3 cups chopped fresh tomatoes or 1 16-ounce can low-
sodium tomatoes
1 cup sliced mushrooms
½ teaspoon dried basil or 2 tablespoons fresh
6 cups Basic Chicken Stock, defatted (see index for recipe)

Combine all ingredients in a large pot. Bring to a boil and simmer, covered, for 1 hour or until rice is completely cooked.

VARIATION

Use barley or other grain in place of rice. Add additional vegetables as desired.

MAKES 6 SERVINGS

calories per serving	110	carbohydrate	22 g (80%)
cholesterol	0	sodium	32 mg
fat	.6 g (5%)	caloric density	27
protein	3 g (11%)		

MINESTRONE

½ *cup chopped onion*
½ *cup chopped celery*
1 clove garlic, minced
3 cups Basic Chicken or Beef Stock, defatted (see index for recipe)
1 16-ounce can low-sodium tomatoes, chopped
2 tablespoons chopped parsley
2 teaspoons dried basil, crushed
1 teaspoon dried oregano, crushed
1 bay leaf
1 cup diced potatoes, uncooked
1 cup sliced carrots
¾ *cup canned red kidney beans, rinsed and drained*
½ *cup whole wheat pasta, uncooked (spaghetti or elbow)*
2 tablespoons sapsago cheese (optional)

1. *In large saucepan, cook onion, celery, and garlic in small amount of stock until tender but not brown. Stir in remainder of broth, undrained tomatoes, parsley, basil, oregano, and bay leaf.*

2. *Simmer, covered, for 30 minutes. Add potatoes and carrots; simmer, covered, about 15 minutes or until vegetables are tender. Add beans and pasta. Cook 15 minutes more or until pasta is tender, stirring occasionally.*

3. *Remove bay leaf. Pour soup into bowls and sprinkle each serving with small amounts of sapsago cheese for garnish (optional).*

VARIATION

Combine all ingredients except pasta. Bring to boil; reduce heat and simmer for 45 minutes. Add pasta and cook 15 minutes longer.

MAKES 4 SERVINGS

calories per serving	200	carbohydrate	40 g (80%)
cholesterol	0	sodium	200 mg
fat	.7 g (3%)	caloric density	43
protein	8 g (16%)		

CHICKEN AND CHILI SOUP

6 cups Basic Chicken Stock, defatted (see index for recipe)
2 cups green beans, fresh or frozen
2 medium carrots, cut into ¼-inch-round chunks
1 small tomato, peeled, seeded and chopped
1 cup cooked or canned garbanzo beans, rinsed and drained
1 tablespoon dried cilantro or parsley or 2 tablespoons
  chopped fresh
2 canned green chilies, rinsed and drained
1 cup cooked and shredded chicken (white breast meat)
6 lime wedges

1. Heat chicken stock to boil. Add green beans, carrots, and tomatoes and cook for approximately 20 minutes or until tender.

2. Add garbanzo beans, cilantro, and chilies and cook for 5 minutes more. Remove chilies and tear into strips.

3. Place a small amount of chicken and chili strips in each bowl. Top with soup. Serve with lime wedge on the side.

VARIATION

Cook all ingredients together for approximately 30 minutes. Add shredded corn tortillas to soup during last 5 minutes of cooking.

MAKES 6 SERVINGS

calories per serving	155	carbohydrate	20 g (52%)
cholesterol	24 mg	sodium	57 mg
fat	2 g (11%)	caloric density	41
protein	14 g (36%)		

FESTIVE SOUP

2 potatoes, diced
2 onions, minced
2 cloves garlic, minced
2 green chilies, seeded and minced
2 tablespoons Basic Chicken Stock, defatted (see index for recipe)
1 leek, washed and chopped
1 teaspoon paprika
5 cups Basic Chicken Stock, defatted (see index for recipe)
⅓ cup dry red wine
2 tomatoes, chopped
Dash ground cloves (optional)

1. *Sauté potatoes, onions, garlic, and chilies in 2 tablespoons chicken stock over medium-low heat in a large nonstick pot or kettle (or use small amount of vegetable spray over bottom before adding ingredients). Cook 5 minutes, stirring often, until potatoes are lightly browned.*
2. *Add leek and cook 3 minutes more, stirring frequently.*
3. *Add paprika, 5 cups defatted chicken stock, and wine. Cook 10 minutes, continuing to stir. Add tomatoes. Cook 15 minutes, stirring occasionally. Add dash of cloves (optional).*

MAKES 8 SERVINGS

calories per serving	83	carbohydrate	18 g (86%)
cholesterol	0	sodium	26.0 mg
fat	.3 g (3%)	caloric density	24
protein	2 g (10%)		

GAZPACHO

Serve this soup cold or hot.

2 16-ounce cans low-sodium tomatoes or **2 pounds large fresh
tomatoes, peeled**
½ cucumber, peeled and seeded
½ bell pepper, seeded
1 large red onion, chopped
1 clove garlic, minced
2 tablespoons red wine vinegar
Dash hot pepper sauce (Tabasco)
Dash freshly ground pepper (optional)
1 12-ounce can low-sodium tomato juice
⅓ cup chopped chives
Yogurt and chopped green or red pepper or scallions (garnish)

1. *Combine all ingredients except chives and garnish in food processor or blender. Puree for a smoother soup or pulse for a chunky vegetable style.*

2. *Chill for several hours. Serve in individual chilled bowls. Sprinkle
chives on top with a dollop of nonfat yogurt. Also, top soup with green or
red pepper or scallions for garnish.*

VARIATION

*For a quick method of chilling, add ice cubes to soup, cover, and chill
for 20 minutes, stirring occasionally.*

MAKES 6 SERVINGS

calories per serving	70	carbohydrate	16 g (91%)
cholesterol	0	sodium	35 mg
fat	.1 g (1%)	caloric density	26
protein	1 g (6%)		

LENTIL SOUP

1 cup dried lentils
1 medium onion, chopped
1 clove garlic, minced
2 medium carrots, diced
1 medium celery stalk, chopped
1 small potato, uncooked, diced
1 bay leaf
⅛ teaspoon dry mustard
⅛ teaspoon cayenne pepper (or more to taste)
4 cups Basic Chicken Stock, defatted, (see index for recipe) or
*   water*
Freshly ground pepper (optional)

1. *Combine all ingredients except pepper in a large pot. Cover and bring to boil. Simmer for 1½–2 hours or until lentils are very tender. Stir occasionally. Add ground pepper to taste.*

2. *To thicken soup, puree half in a food processor or blender. Return to the pot and cook 5 minutes longer.*

VARIATION

Use split peas in place of lentils.

Makes 4 Servings

calories per serving	115	carbohydrate	22 g (76%)
cholesterol	0	sodium	43 mg
fat	.2 g (1%)	caloric density	44
protein	7 g (23%)		

QUICK CORN CHOWDER

½ cup Basic Chicken Stock, defatted, (see index for recipe) or
  water
2 cups corn kernels, fresh or frozen
1½ cups nonfat milk (liquid)
2 teaspoons dried onion flakes
⅛ teaspoon garlic powder
½ teaspoon chili salsa
2 teaspoons lemon juice
1 tablespoon cornstarch
¼ cup cold water
½ teaspoon paprika

1. Place stock and corn in a pot and bring to boil. Drain corn, reserving stock. Put one-half of the corn into blender or food processor with milk, onion flakes, garlic powder, salsa, and lemon juice. Blend 10 seconds.

2. Pour soup back into saucepan with remaining corn and simmer on low.

3. Add 1 tablespoon cornstarch to ¼ cup cold water; mix until smooth and pour into soup. Cook for 2 minutes or until heated, constantly stirring. To serve, sprinkle with paprika.

VARIATIONS

1. Add ½ cup cooked scallops, clams, or oysters.
2. Add a diced potato in place of cornstarch.

MAKES 4 SERVINGS

calories per serving	133	carbohydrate	26 g (78%)
cholesterol	1.5 mg	sodium	52 mg
fat	1 g (6%)	caloric density	62
protein	5 g (15%)		

ORIENTAL VEGETABLE SOUP

4 cups Basic Chicken Stock, defatted (see index for recipe)
1 cup fresh bean sprouts
⅔ cup fresh snow peas or 1 6-ounce package frozen snow peas,
  thawed
⅓ cup sliced scallions or green onions
2 tablespoons dry sherry
1 teaspoon garlic powder
1 teaspoon apple juice concentrate, thawed
1 teaspoon low-sodium soy sauce
5 egg whites

In large saucepan, over medium-high heat, combine stock, bean sprouts, and snow peas. Bring to boil; reduce heat to simmer and cook, covered, for 2 minutes. Add scallions, sherry, garlic powder, apple juice, and soy sauce, one at a time, stirring after each addition. Without stirring, slowly add egg whites. Cook for 30 seconds. Stir twice.

VARIATIONS

1. Add ½ cup cooked and diced chicken or turkey.
2. Steam 4 ounces of fish in chicken broth. Add with other ingredients.
3. For a vegetarian version, add 4 ounces diced tofu.

MAKES 5 SERVINGS

calories per serving	59	carbohydrate	9 g (61%)
cholesterol	0	sodium	92 mg
fat	.1 g (1%)	caloric density	33
protein	4 g (27%)		

15
SALADS AND VEGETABLES: COLORFUL KEYS TO HEALTH

The beauty of vegetables deserves special attention. Their coolness, crispness, and great nutritional benefits make them irresistible. Enticing combinations of ingredients add elegance and zest to the basic menu. Vegetables are truly an asset to your eating plan. The high fiber content of vegetables encourages you to fill up with an abundance of vitamins and minerals with very few calories. In addition to the benefit of weight loss, studies have supported the important role certain vegetables play in reducing the risk of heart disease and some forms of cancer because of their soluble fiber components.

Unfortunately, most Americans eat vegetables grudgingly, consuming them infrequently. Of course, it is the method of preparing vegetables (overcooking in huge pots of water) that makes the flavors a penance rather than a pleasure. Full flavors are preserved when you learn to cook vegetables properly.

This chapter provides guidelines for selecting, storing, and preparing vegetables properly and for maintaining quality taste and nutrient appeal. Recipes are included for cold salads, warm cooked salads, and vegetable dishes to be served on the side or as the main course.

GUIDELINES FOR VEGETABLES

1. Always include a variety of fresh vegetables on your shopping list to obtain the most flavor in your recipes. Frozen vegetables can be purchased and kept on hand for preparing "quick" dishes. Look for unsalted frozen vegetables. In general, it is best to avoid canned vegetables, which usually contain salt and sugar and lack flavor. Occasional use of canned vegetables or other products in recipes is acceptable. However, be sure to rinse and drain the contents of the can before using.

2. When cooking vegetables, use as little water as possible. The preferred cooking method for retaining nutrients and maintaining the crispness and color of vegetables is to steam, stir-fry, or blanch. Save any left-over liquid and use in soups, casseroles, sauces, stocks, or for cooking grains.

3. Vegetables can be frozen after cooking in an airtight sealed container. Avoid freezing raw vegetables.

4. Include a variety of vegetables in your diet. Avoid boredom by experimenting with exotic or seasonal types. Also, select different forms of vegetables within the same family. For example, there are many kinds of cabbages with distinctly different flavors that you can try working with.

5. When storing vegetables, prevent excessive exposure to water, air, heat, or light. Most vegetables should be kept in the refrigerator to prevent spoilage. Other vegetables such as those in the potato family (potatoes, yams, and sweet potatoes) should be stored in a cool, dark area. Avoid storing potatoes in the refrigerator, which breaks down the starches to sugars and affects the flavor of the potato.

6. Have on hand a large container of cut-up raw vegetables to munch on. These can be prepared in advance and placed in a bowl with ice to keep them well preserved.

TOMATO BASIL SALAD

4 medium tomatoes, sliced thin
1 small red onion, sliced thin
¼ cup fresh basil or 2 teaspoons dried basil
¼–⅓ cup red wine vinegar
Freshly ground pepper to taste

1. *Layer tomatoes and onion and sprinkle with basil.*
2. *Pour vinegar over salad and add pepper if desired. Marinate for 1 to 2 hours in refrigerator. Add more pepper to taste when serving.*

VARIATIONS

1. *Add sliced cucumber.*
2. *To create a spicy flavor, use a dash hot pepper sauce (Tabasco).*

MAKES 5 SERVINGS

calories per serving	39	carbohydrate	8 g (82%)
cholesterol	0	sodium	5 mg
fat	.3 g (7%)	caloric density	24
protein	1 g (10%)		

ITALIAN DELIGHT

6 cups torn spinach leaves
1 cup sliced radishes
1 small green pepper, cut into strips
1 cup shredded carrots
1 cup fresh tomato wedges
2–3 tablespoons sapsago cheese (optional)

In a large bowl, combine all ingredients; toss to coat with any L.A. Diet salad dressing.

VARIATION

Use dark green lettuce in place of spinach.

Makes 6 Servings

calories per serving	26	carbohydrate	5 g (77%)
cholesterol	0	sodium	5 mg
fat	.2 g (6%)	caloric density	29
protein	1 g (15%)		

CUCUMBERS VINAIGRETTE

2 medium cucumbers, peeled and sliced
3 green onions, sliced thin
⅛ teaspoon dried tarragon, crushed
2 tablespoons unsweetened pineapple juice concentrate
½ cup unsweetened rice vinegar

Combine all ingredients. Marinate for several hours in refrigerator. Drain and serve.

VARIATION

Add diced red pepper for color.

MAKES 8 SERVINGS

calories per serving	16	carbohydrate	3 g (75%)
cholesterol	0	sodium	3 mg
fat	.1 g (5%)	caloric density	25
protein	.5 g (12%)		

SUPREME GARDEN SALAD

3 cups salad greens
3 small tomatoes, diced
4 green onions, sliced thin
1 cucumber, diced
6 radishes, sliced thin
3 hard-cooked egg whites, chopped
½ cup nonfat dry-curd cottage cheese, crumbled
1 cup cut-up cooked chicken or turkey (in strips)

Combine all vegetables. Sprinkle with egg whites and cheese. Top with chicken or turkey strips.

MAKES 6 SERVINGS

calories per serving	76	carbohydrate	6 g (32%)
cholesterol	15 mg	sodium	33 mg
fat	1 g (11%)	caloric density	71
protein	10 g (52%)		

TOMATO RICE SALAD

1 tablespoon low-sodium soy sauce
1 tablespoon red wine vinegar or rice vinegar (for milder
flavor)
3 cups cooked and cooled long-grain brown rice
3 medium tomatoes, seeded and diced
1 green pepper, seeded and diced
½ red onion, diced
2 tablespoons chopped fresh basil or 1 tablespoon dried basil

1. Sprinkle soy sauce and vinegar over rice. Mix lightly with fork.
2. Add tomatoes, green pepper, red onion, and basil. Toss lightly.
3. Chill until serving time.

VARIATIONS

1. Add diced pimiento or red pepper.
2. Serve warm instead of cold.

MAKES 8 SERVINGS

calories per serving	101	carbohydrate	22 g (87%)
cholesterol	0	sodium	132 mg
fat	.6 g (5%)	caloric density	71
protein	2 g (8%)		

BROCCOLI PASTA SALAD

4 cups broccoli spears
½ cup sliced mushrooms
1 cup cooked eggless pasta (spiral-shaped)
2 tablespoons rinsed and drained pimientos
Italian Vinaigrette

1. Steam broccoli and mushrooms until lightly cooked but not
tender. Cool to room temperature.
2. In a bowl, combine vegetables with cooked pasta and pimientos.
Splash on Italian dressing and toss lightly. Chill before serving.

VARIATIONS

1. *Add red pepper in place of pimientos.*
2. *Serve warm instead of cold.*

Makes 8 Servings

calories per serving	50	carbohydrate	8 g (69%)
cholesterol	0	sodium	9 mg
fat	.4 g (7%)	caloric density	41
protein	3 g (24%)		

SPECIAL SPINACH SALAD

4 cups salad greens (any dark green lettuce)
4 cups torn spinach
1 medium orange, sliced and sectioned
1 8-ounce can water chestnuts, drained and sliced
1 cup sliced mushrooms
1 small red onion, sliced and separated into rings
½ cup seeded and diced red pepper

In large bowl, combine all ingredients except dressing. Chill until serving time. Toss with any L.A. Diet salad dressing.

VARIATION

Use 1 11-ounce can Mandarin oranges, drained, in place of fresh orange.

Makes 6 Servings

calories per serving	50	carbohydrate	10 g (80%)
cholesterol	0	sodium	14 mg
fat	.2 g (4%)	caloric density	36
protein	2 g (16%)		

SUNSHINE FRUIT AND YOGURT SALAD

Wake up your morning with this beautiful and tasty salad!

1 medium golden delicious or green Granny Smith apple,
   cubed
1 medium red delicious apple, cubed
½ cup seedless green grapes
1 medium orange, sectioned
½ cup chopped celery
1 cup sliced banana (1 large)
1 tablespoon raisins or diced dates

Dressing

½ cup plain nonfat yogurt
¼ teaspoon ground cinnamon
1 teaspoon unsweetened apple or pineapple juice concentrate

Paprika and Grapenuts (for garnish)

1. *In large bowl, combine all ingredients except dressing.*
2. *To make dressing, whisk together yogurt, cinnamon, and apple or pineapple juice concentrate. Toss with salad. Garnish with paprika and top each serving with 1 teaspoon Grapenuts (optional).*

VARIATIONS

1. *Add any combination of fruit in season.*
2. *To make spicy, add a small dash of cayenne pepper.*

MAKES 4 SERVINGS

calories per serving	138	carbohydrate	31 g (90%)
cholesterol	.5 mg	sodium	36 mg
fat	.7 g (4%)	caloric density	70
protein	2 g (6%)		

SWEET 'N' SOUR CARROT SALAD

6 large carrots, peeled and grated
½ cup raisins
1 medium green apple, unpeeled and grated

Dressing

½ cup plain nonfat yogurt
1 tablespoon lemon juice
1 tablespoon unseasoned rice vinegar

1. *In large bowl, combine carrots, raisins, and apple.*
2. *Separately, mix ingredients for dressing until smooth. Toss salad and dressing together.*

VARIATION

Soak raisins in lemon juice or orange juice until plump. Add to salad.

MAKES 6 SERVINGS

calories per serving	104	carbohydrate	23 g (88%)
cholesterol	0	sodium	63 mg
fat	.4 g (3%)	caloric density	68
protein	2 g (7%)		

ORIENTAL CUCUMBER SALAD

2 cups thinly sliced peeled cucumbers
½ cup chopped green onions

Dressing

¼ cup unseasoned rice vinegar
1 tablespoon unsweetened apple juice concentrate
2 teaspoons low-sodium soy sauce
1 clove fresh garlic, crushed

Sliced tomatoes for garnish

1. *In large bowl, combine cucumbers and onions.*
2. *Combine ingredients for dressing. Splash over vegetables. Refrigerate before serving. Garnish with sliced tomatoes.*

VARIATIONS

1. *Add diced red pepper.*
2. *Double or triple salad dressing and use to marinate chicken or fish.*

MAKES 4 SERVINGS

calories per serving	25	carbohydrate	5 g (80%)
cholesterol	0	sodium	151 mg
fat	.2 g (7%)	caloric density	30
protein	.7 g (11%)		

SNOW PEA AND PASTA SALAD

6 ounces whole wheat pasta (eggless, any shape), uncooked
1 small onion, chopped
1 clove garlic, minced
3 tablespoons Basic Chicken Stock, defatted (see index for recipe)
1 15-ounce can garbanzo beans, rinsed and drained
¼ cup white wine vinegar
1 teaspoon unsweetened apple juice concentrate
1 teaspoon minced, fresh oregano leaf or ½ teaspoon dried oregano
⅛ teaspoon freshly ground black pepper
1 cup broccoli flowerets, steamed
1 6-ounce package frozen snow peas, thawed, or ⅔ cup fresh, steamed
2 tablespoons pimiento, rinsed and drained
Romaine or other leafy green lettuce (garnish)

1. Following package directions, cook pasta to al dente; drain, rinse with cold water, drain again, and reserve.

2. Using a nonstick skillet, sauté onion and garlic in chicken stock for 3 minutes or until tender. Avoid browning. Remove with slotted spoon to large bowl.

3. Stir in beans, vinegar, apple juice, oregano, and pepper, mixing well.

4. Add broccoli and snow peas, mixing well. Add pasta and pimiento; toss lightly. (Avoid tearing pasta by overmixing.) Cover; refrigerate 4 hours or overnight.

5. To serve, line salad bowl with lettuce leafs; place pasta salad over lettuce.

VARIATION

Add 1 cup halved cherry tomatoes.

MAKES 6 SERVINGS

calories per serving	274	carbohydrate	52 g (76%)
cholesterol	0	sodium	6 mg
fat	2 g (6%)	caloric density	108
protein	13 g (18%)		

CHINESE CHICKEN SALAD

4 cups finely shredded Chinese cabbage
⅛ cup chopped scallions or green onions
½ cup mung bean sprouts
¼ cup sliced mushrooms
¼ cup sliced carrot (1 medium)
½ medium tomato, sliced
⅛ cup raisins
⅛ cup thinly sliced green pepper
1 medium celery stalk, sliced thin
½ cup cut-up cooked white chicken breast (in strips)

Dressing

¼ cup unseasoned rice vinegar
1 tablespoon unsweetened apple juice concentrate
2 teaspoons low-sodium soy sauce

1. *In large bowl, combine all ingredients except dressing and toss.*
2. *Prepare dressing in separate container and mix. Splash over salad. Refrigerate before serving.*

VARIATIONS

1. *Add ½ cup cooked fish such as salmon, scallops, or any white fish in place of chicken.*
2. *Add any favorite vegetable.*
3. *The fish or chicken can be warmed before adding to salad.*

MAKES 2 SERVINGS

calories per serving	83	carbohydrate	15 g (72%)
cholesterol	11 mg	sodium	137 mg
fat	1 g (11%)	caloric density	47
protein	3 g (14%)		

SALMON SALAD

1 8-ounce can red sockeye salmon, rinsed and drained
½ cup unsweetened orange juice
¼ cup freshly squeezed lemon juice
1 medium cucumber, peeled and chopped
1 medium green pepper, halved, seeded, and chopped
½ medium red pepper, halved, seeded, and minced
1 medium tomato, peeled, cored, seeded, and chopped
½ medium red onion, pared and minced
3 tablespoons minced green onion (green tops only)
Dark green lettuce
Cherry tomatoes and 1 tablespoon chopped fresh parsley (for
garnish)
Lime wedges

1. *Bone salmon, break into bite-size pieces, and place in bowl. Combine orange and lemon juices and pour over salmon.*

2. *Combine cucumber, green and red peppers, tomato, and red and green onions in bowl.*

3. *Add one-third of vegetable mixture to salmon, mixing gently. Cover both bowls and refrigerate 3–4 hours.*

4. *At serving time, arrange salmon mixture on bed of lettuce in salad bowl. Place reserved vegetables over salmon. Garnish with cherry tomatoes and parsley. Serve with lime wedges.*

VARIATION

Use 1 7-ounce can water-packed tuna in place of salmon.

MAKES 8 SERVINGS

calories per serving	81	carbohydrate	6 g (30%)
cholesterol	10 mg	sodium	107 mg
fat	3 g (34%)	caloric density	75
protein	7 g (34%)		

REFRESHING PINEAPPLE SALAD FOR ONE

2 unsweetened, canned pineapple slices
Romaine lettuce leaves
½ cup 1 percent low-fat cottage cheese rinsed and drained
Dash paprika (garnish)

Place pineapple rings on romaine lettuce. Top with cottage cheese. Sprinkle with paprika for garnish.

VARIATION

Substitute peaches or pears for the pineapple.

Makes 1 Serving

calories per serving	157	carbohydrate	23 g (58%)
cholesterol	2 mg	sodium	46 mg
fat	1 g (6%)	caloric density	66
protein	14 g (36%)		

BASIC GREEN GARDEN SALAD

4 cups dark green lettuce
1 large tomato, sliced
½ cup sliced cucumber (½ medium)
⅓ cup garbanzo or other beans, rinsed and drained

Dressing

½ cup balsamic vinegar or red wine vinegar
1 tablespoon dried tarragon, crushed, or 2 tablespoons fresh
   tarragon leaves

Chives and freshly ground black pepper (garnish)

1. *In large bowl, combine vegetables and beans.*
2. *Combine dressing ingredients and toss with salad. Sprinkle chives and black pepper over salad to garnish.*

VARIATIONS

1. *Add any raw vegetables of your choice.*
2. *Use an Italian dressing without oil in place of red wine vinegar mixture.*

MAKES 4 SERVINGS

calories per serving	74	carbohydrate	14 g (75%)
cholesterol	0	sodium	6 mg
fat	.8 g (9%)	caloric density	48
protein	3 g (16%)		

CHILLED VEGETABLE-RICE SALAD

2 cups cooked and chilled long-grain brown rice
1½ cups corn kernels, fresh or frozen, thawed
1 cup celery chunks
1 cup grated carrot
2 medium green onions, chopped

Combine all ingredients and toss in a dressing of your choice.

VARIATION

Add 1½ cups green peas.

MAKES 4 SERVINGS

calories per serving	196	carbohydrate	43 g (87%)
cholesterol	0	sodium	87 mg
fat	1 g (2%)	caloric density	86
protein	5 g (10%)		

CREAMY PASTA PRIMAVERA

10 ounces eggless whole wheat pasta, uncooked
½ cup diced celery
¼ cup diced green pepper
½ cup sliced fresh mushrooms
½ cup diced onion
1 medium tomato, diced
¼ cup chopped pimiento
1 cup broccoli flowerets
¼ cup Basic Chicken Stock (see index for recipe)

Dressing

1 cup Grazing Cream Cheese (see index for recipe) or 1 percent
  low-fat cottage cheese, rinsed and drained
2 teaspoons lemon juice
1 teaspoon dry mustard
1 tablespoon Worcestershire sauce
1 teaspoon unsweetened apple juice concentrate
½ teaspoon paprika
Freshly ground pepper

½ cup tomato, quartered (garnish)

1. *Cook pasta according to package directions. Drain well and rinse with cool water. Set aside.*

2. *In a large skillet over medium heat, sauté celery, green pepper, mushrooms, onion, diced tomato, pimiento, and broccoli in ¼ cup chicken stock until vegetables are crisp but not overcooked. Drain liquid. Remove from heat and allow to cool to room temperature. Place in refrigerator until ready to add dressing.*

3. *Prepare dressing by blending ingredients for 2 to 3 minutes in a blender until smooth and creamy.*

4. *Fold dressing into vegetables. Add cooked pasta and mix until well coated. Garnish with tomato quarters.*

VARIATIONS

1. Use no-oil Italian or vinaigrette dressing in place of the creamy dressing.

2. Add diced fish if desired.

3. Serve leftovers as a cold salad and stuff into tomatoes or peppers.

MAKES 10 SERVINGS

calories per serving	174	carbohydrate	35 g (80%)
cholesterol	1 mg	sodium	23 mg
fat	1 g (5%)	caloric density	80
protein	8 g (18%)		

WARM SQUASH AND ONION SALAD

1 small onion sliced thin
1 clove garlic, minced
¼ cup white wine
1 pound yellow squash, sliced ¼ inch thick
2 tablespoons water
Freshly ground pepper (optional)

1. Cook and stir onion and garlic in white wine in large nonstick skillet over medium heat for 4 minutes or until tender.

2. Add squash and water. Cover tightly and continue cooking 7 minutes or until squash is crisp-tender. Season with freshly ground pepper or other herb (optional).

VARIATION

Use zucchini in place of squash or a combination of the two.

MAKES 4 SERVINGS

calories per serving	47	carbohydrate	10 g (85%)
cholesterol	0	sodium	4 mg
fat	.2 g (3%)	caloric density	21
protein	1 g (8%)		

BALSAMIC POTATO SALAD

2 pounds red new potatoes, cut into chunks
1 cup plain nonfat yogurt
¼ cup balsamic vinegar
1 cup sliced scallions
2 teaspoons low-sodium soy sauce
1 tablespoon unsweetened apple juice concentrate
1 tablespoon dried dill or 2 tablespoons fresh dill
1½ cups coarsely chopped celery
½ cup sliced radishes
½ cup diced red delicious apple
Romaine lettuce leaves (garnish)
Dash paprika (garnish)

1. Cook potatoes in a large pot of boiling water over medium-high heat until tender (15–20 minutes). Drain potatoes in a strainer or colander. Transfer to a bowl and cool.

2. In a separate bowl, combine yogurt, vinegar, scallions, soy sauce, apple juice, and dill and whisk until smooth.

3. Once potatoes have cooled, add dressing. Toss to coat.

4. Add celery, radishes, and apple to potatoes and toss to combine. Line serving bowl with lettuce. Place potato salad over lettuce and sprinkle with paprika for garnish.

VARIATION

Use 2 pounds of vegetables of your choice in place of potatoes.

MAKES 12 SERVINGS

calories per serving	67	carbohydrate	14 g (83%)
cholesterol	1 mg	sodium	65 mg
fat	.4 g (5%)	caloric density	59
protein	2 g (12%)		

16
SAUCES, DRESSINGS, AND DIPS: FLAVOR WITHOUT COMPROMISE

A special sauce or dressing can make the difference between a great meal and one that is mediocre. The flavor, color, and texture provided by a lovely glaze or salad dressing are wonderful additions to a favorite poached fish, a steaming bowl of rice, or a cold, crisp bowl of fruit. You can use the recipes in this chapter to flavor just about anything.

The following pages provide recipes for sauces, glazes, dressings, and dips. Guidelines and tips are presented to help make the most of this special part of your menu. Whether for a special occasion or an everyday meal, these low-fat, low-cholesterol, and low-calorie additions can add flavor to your food without compromise.

GUIDELINES FOR PREPARING SAUCES, DRESSINGS, AND DIPS

1. To thicken sauce, use cornstarch, arrowroot, masa (derived from corn), or whole wheat flour. To prevent lumps, be sure to add thickener to a liquid that is cold or at room temperature before adding to a heated saucepan.
2. For a thin sauce, prepare the base with defatted chicken stock or another acceptable liquid. Add additional liquid until desired consistency is achieved. To make a creamy sauce, add nonfat milk powder.
3. Use various herbs, spices, and condiments such as Worcestershire sauce, unsalted mustard, wine, apple juice, or tomato paste to create flavor for a sauce, dressing, or dip.
4. To prepare salad dressings, use a vinegar base such as rice vinegar (unseasoned), balsamic vinegar, red wine vinegar, or raspberry vinegar and add other ingredients to provide specific flavor combinations. To reduce acidity in a salad dressing, use balsamic or rice vinegar, which tend to be lower in acid content than the average red or white vinegar.
5. Whenever possible, use unsalted ingredients such as mustards and tomato products. These condiments have significantly lower sodium levels.
6. Avoid commercially bottled "low-calorie" salad dressings that contain oil, sugar, and salt.
7. To create creaminess in dips, use a product that provides a cream base such as nonfat dry-curd cottage cheese, 1 percent low-fat cottage cheese, nonfat yogurt, nonfat milk powder, or tofu. When using 1 percent low-fat cottage cheese, be sure to rinse under cold water and drain. This helps remove the cream, a source of fat. Cream in a blender or food processor until smooth. Whenever working with nonfat dry-curd cottage cheese, be sure to blend by itself before adding additional ingredients. This prevents a grainy texture from forming.

8. Use the peel from a lemon, orange, or Mandarin orange to add zesty flavor to a sauce or glaze. Fresh or frozen fruit can be added to sweeten a sauce or glaze.

9. A blender or food processor can be used to mix and combine ingredients. A hand mixer can also assist in combining thicker ingredients. Most dressings can be prepared and combined by hand using a wire whisk.

10. Sauces, dressings, and dips can be served cold or warm, depending on the recipe. For example, a warm sweet glaze is a nice addition over fruit, or a chilled dressing can provide flavor to a crisp salad.

11. Store in tightly closed jar in refrigerator.

We'll begin with a selection of both sweet and savory cheese spreads that add a nice filling and flavor to a basic bread, bagel, or baked good. Also, these cheese spreads can be prepared as dips to be served with fruit, vegetables, or crackers. Dressings and sauces will follow to help you add some spice, flavor, and fun to your food!

BASIC GRAZING CREAM CHEESE

1 pound nonfat dry-curd cottage cheese or 1 percent low-fat
cottage cheese, rinsed and drained
½ cup skim milk
1 tablespoon plain nonfat yogurt

1. *Blend cottage cheese in food processor or blender until it forms a ball or adheres to the sides of the container.*
2. *Add remaining ingredients and blend until smooth.*

MAKES 16 SERVINGS

calories per serving	43	carbohydrate	2 g (19%)
cholesterol	2 mg	sodium	25 mg
fat	.6 g (13%)	caloric density	68
protein	7 g (65%)		

VARIATIONS

To the Basic Grazing Cream Cheese, you can add any combination of ingredients to provide a specific flavor. Try some of the following variations and use as dips, sandwich fillings, or "cheese" to spread on toast.

1. Banana Cream Cheese: *After step 1, add 1 ripe banana, ⅓ cup unsweetened apple juice concentrate, and 1 tablespoon vanilla and blend.*

2. Date and Raisin Cheese: *After step 1, add ½ cup pitted dates and ½ cup raisins and blend.*

3. Savory Cream Cheese: *After step 1, add 1 10-ounce package frozen mixed vegetables (thawed), 2 tablespoons Worcestershire sauce, dash each garlic powder and onion powder, and 1 teaspoon low-sodium soy sauce.*

4. Spinach Cheese: *After step 1, add 1 10-ounce package frozen spinach (thawed and drained), dash each garlic and onion powder, 2 tablespoons Worcestershire sauce, and 3 ounces diced green chilies (rinsed).*

YOGURT CHEESE

2 cups plain nonfat yogurt

1. *Place a hand strainer over a bowl and line with 1 generous piece of triple-layer cheesecloth. Place yogurt in cheesecloth-lined strainer. Wrap yogurt with cloth and place in the refrigerator overnight.*

2. *The next day, unwrap the yogurt. Place yogurt-cheese in closed container and store up to 3 weeks in the refrigerator. Do not freeze the cheese.*

To reduce tartness, add 2–3 tablespoons nonfat milk powder to the yogurt in step 1 and mix well.

MAKES 16 SERVINGS

calories per serving	8	carbohydrate	1 g (50%)
cholesterol	0.2 mg	sodium	11 mg
fat	0.02 g (2%)	caloric density	56
protein	0.8 g (40%)		

VARIATIONS

To the Yogurt Cheese recipe, you can add various ingredients to create a thick, flavored cheese spread. Try the following suggestions.

1. Pineapple Yogurt Cheese Spread: *In step 1, add 1 cup unsweetened crushed pineapple, drained, and mix well.*

2. Spicy Yogurt Cheese Spread: *In step 1, add 3 ounces diced green chilies, rinsed and drained, 1–2 drops Tabasco sauce, and dash garlic powder; mix well.*

3. Dill Yogurt Cheese Spread: *In step 1, add 3 tablespoons fresh dill or 4 teaspoons dried dill, 1–2 diced green onions, and 1–2 tablespoons diced pimientos, rinsed and drained; mix well into yogurt.*

4. Onion Yogurt Cheese Spread: *In step 1, add 2 tablespoons dehydrated onion flakes, 1 tablespoon dried parsley flakes, and dash garlic powder to yogurt and mix well. Garnish with chives.*

BASIC GRAZING SOUR CREAM

1–2 teaspoons lemon juice
½ cup skim milk
1 pound nonfat dry-curd cottage cheese or 1 percent low-fat
  cottage cheese, rinsed and drained

1. Add lemon juice to skim milk and let stand for 1–2 minutes until milk curdles and forms a buttermilk consistency.
2. Blend cottage cheese in a food processor or blender until cheese forms a ball or adheres to the sides of the container. Add milk a little at a time until the desired consistency is formed.

VARIATION

Add 1 tablespoon plain nonfat yogurt along with the milk for a tangy flavor.

MAKES 16 SERVINGS

calories per serving	43	carbohydrate	2 g (18%)
cholesterol	2 mg	sodium	25 mg
fat	0.6 g (13%)	caloric density	68
protein	7 g (65%)		

SALAD DRESSINGS

BASIC CREAMY SALAD DRESSING

Use this salad dressing as a substitute for mayonnaise.

1 cup nonfat dry-curd cottage cheese or 1 percent low-fat
  cottage cheese, rinsed and drained
2 egg whites
¼ cup unseasoned rice vinegar
1 tablespoon unsalted Dijon mustard
1 teaspoon Italian herbs
1 tablespoon chopped fresh parsley (garnish)

  Blend cottage cheese in food processor or blender until cheese adheres to the sides of the container. Add remaining ingredients except parsley and blend until smooth. Garnish with parsley.

VARIATION

  For a tangy flavor, add ¼ cup plain nonfat yogurt.

MAKES 8 SERVINGS

calories per serving	45	carbohydrate	2 g (26%)
cholesterol	2 mg	sodium	5 mg
fat	.2 g (6%)	caloric density	66
protein	5 g (66%)		

SHERRY GARLIC DRESSING

½ cup water
1 cup dry sherry
2 cloves fresh garlic, minced
1 teaspoon dry mustard
2 tablespoons unsweetened apple juice concentrate
1 tablespoon Worcestershire sauce
1 tablespoon cornstarch
¼ cup water

1. *Place all ingredients except cornstarch and ¼ cup water together in a saucepan. Bring to boil; reduce heat, cover, and simmer for 10 minutes.*

2. *Dissolve cornstarch in ¼ cup water until smooth. Add to saucepan and continue to cook until slightly thickened. Serve hot or cold.*

VARIATION

For a ginger flavor, add 2 tablespoons grated fresh gingerroot or 1 teaspoon dried.

MAKES 12 SERVINGS

calories per serving	15	carbohydrate	3 g (80%)
cholesterol	0 mg	sodium	13 mg
fat	.05 g (3%)	caloric density	60
protein	.2 g (6%)		

THOUSAND ISLAND DRESSING

1 cup Grazing Sour Cream (see index for recipe)
2 drops Worcestershire sauce
¼ teaspoon finely grated onion
1 hard-cooked egg white, chopped
1 tablespoon tomato paste
2 teaspoons finely chopped fresh parsley
Dash freshly ground black pepper

Combine all ingredients in a blender or food processor.

VARIATIONS

1. *Add 1 tablespoon lemon juice for a sharper tangy flavor.*
2. *To thin the dressing, add skim milk until desired consistency is achieved.*

MAKES 10 SERVINGS

calories per serving	18	carbohydrate	1 g (22%)
cholesterol	.9 mg	sodium	10 mg
fat	.1 g (5%)	caloric density	66
protein	3 g (68%)		

ORIENTAL SALAD DRESSING

¼ *cup unseasoned rice wine vinegar*
1 tablespoon unsweetened pineapple juice concentrate
1 tablespoon Worcestershire sauce
Dash garlic and onion powder
Grated fresh gingerroot (optional)
¼ *cup diced green onions*

Mix ingredients together in a bowl. Keep in a jar until ready to use.

VARIATIONS

1. *Double or triple the dressing and use as a marinating base for chicken or fish.*
2. *Splash over hot steamed vegetables.*

MAKES 4 SERVINGS

calories per serving	17	carbohydrate	4 g (94%)
cholesterol	0 mg	sodium	38 mg
fat	.02 g (1%)	caloric density	37
protein	12 g (5%)		

ITALIAN VINAIGRETTE

½ cup red wine vinegar
½ cup water
1 teaspoon low-sodium soy sauce
1 teaspoon garlic powder
1 teaspoon onion powder
1 teaspoon dried basil, crushed
1 teaspoon dried oregano, crushed

Mix all ingredients together. Add to salad and toss.

MAKES 4 SERVINGS

calories per serving	10	carbohydrate	2 g (80%)
cholesterol	0 mg	sodium	50 mg
fat	0 g	caloric density	32
protein	0.3 g (12%)		

CREAMY ITALIAN DRESSING

½ cup Italian Vinaigrette (see recipe above)
1 tablespoon unsalted Dijon mustard
½ cup plain nonfat yogurt or 1 percent low-fat cottage cheese,
  rinsed
1 teaspoon low-sodium soy sauce
2 teaspoons unsweetened apple juice concentrate
Dash Italian herbal blend

Prepare Italian Vinaigrette from recipe above. Combine remaining ingredients and mix well. Add to salad and toss.

VARIATION

To thin the dressing, add small amounts of skim milk or buttermilk.

MAKES 6 SERVINGS

calories per serving	20	carbohydrate	3 g (60%)
cholesterol	0.3 mg	sodium	58 mg
fat	.2 g (9%)	caloric density	53
protein	2 g (20%)		

FRENCH DRESSING

⅔ *cup unseasoned wine vinegar or rice vinegar*
2 tablespoons chopped fresh basil or *1 teaspoon dried*
2 tablespoons chopped fresh parsley or *1 tablespoon dried*
⅓ *cup lemon juice*
½ *teaspoon freshly ground black or white pepper*
2 teaspoons diced lemon rind or peel

   Combine all ingredients in a jar or sealed container. Shake well. Store in refrigerator until ready to use.

MAKES 6 SERVINGS

calories per serving	13	carbohydrate	4 g (92%)
cholesterol	0 mg	sodium	4 mg
fat	.03 g (2%)	caloric density	29
protein	.2 g (6%)		

SAUCES AND GLAZES

BASIC WHITE SAUCE

2 teaspoons nonfat milk powder
1½ cups skim milk
1 tablespoon cornstarch
1 teaspoon low-sodium soy sauce or 1 tablespoon
    Worcestershire sauce
Dash freshly ground black pepper

Combine milk powder with skim milk. Add cornstarch and soy sauce to milk and mix until smooth. Place in a saucepan and bring to boil; stir constantly until thickened. Add pepper; reduce temperature to simmer and continue to stir until desired consistency is achieved.

VARIATIONS

1. Mushroom Sauce: *Add ½ cup finely chopped mushrooms lightly sautéed in wine. Add 2 teaspoons dried parsley as a garnish.*

2. Parsley Sauce: *To 1 cup white sauce, add ¼ cup finely chopped fresh parsley.*

3. "Cheese" Sauce: *To 1 cup white sauce, add ¼ cup nonfat dry-curd cottage cheese or 1 percent low-fat cottage cheese, rinsed and drained, 1 teaspoon low-sodium soy sauce or 1 tablespoon Worcestershire sauce, and dash of black or white pepper. Cook for 5 minutes until thickened and smooth.*

4. Onion-Garlic Sauce: *Sauté ¼ cup chopped onion and 1 crushed fresh garlic clove in wine for 5 minutes. Drain and add to basic white sauce.*

5. Custard: *Omit black pepper and low-sodium soy sauce from the basic white sauce. Add juice and rind of ½ orange, 1 teaspoon vanilla, and 2 tablespoons of raisins.*

MAKES 6 SERVINGS

calories per serving	31	carbohydrate	5 g (65%)
cholesterol	1.0 mg	sodium	30 mg
fat	.05 g (1%)	caloric density	47
protein	2 g (26%)		

TERIYAKI SAUCE OR GLAZE

⅓ *cup Worcestershire sauce*
⅔ *cup water*
2 tablespoons unsweetened apple or pineapple juice
   concentrate
2 cloves fresh garlic, crushed
¼ *teaspoon ground ginger or* ½ *teaspoon fresh*

Combine all ingredients in a jar or container. Store in the refrigerator until ready to use.

VARIATIONS

Reduce water by ⅓ *cup and add* ⅓ *cup sherry or white wine.*

MAKES 8 SERVINGS

calories per serving	17	carbohydrate	4 g (94%)
cholesterol	0	sodium	99 mg
fat	.02 g (1%)	caloric density	67
protein	0.3 g (4%)		

SWEET 'N' SOUR SAUCE

¼ *cup cider vinegar*
¼ *cup unsweetened apple juice concentrate*
¾ *cup pineapple juice, unsweetened*
1 tablespoon unsalted tomato paste
1 tablespoon sherry
½ *teaspoon ground ginger*

   Combine all ingredients in a jar. Shake and store in the refrigerator until ready to use.

Makes 10 Servings

calories per serving	25	carbohydrate	6 g (96%)
cholesterol	0	sodium	3 mg
fat	0	caloric density	47
protein	0.2 g (3%)		

MARINARA SAUCE

8 cloves fresh garlic, minced
4 bay leaves
2 teaspoons dried oregano
2 teaspoons dried basil
2 cups diced onion
1 teaspoon dried parsley
½ *cup red wine*
2 cups sliced mushrooms
2 16-ounce cans low-sodium tomatoes, chopped

   1. In a large skillet, sauté garlic, bay leaves, oregano, basil, onions, and parsley in red wine over medium-low heat. Add mushrooms and simmer, covered, for 5 minutes.
   2. Add tomatoes and continue to simmer, covered, for 30 minutes. Remove bay leaves before serving.

VARIATION

Add 1 cup seafood such as scallops, oysters, calamari (squid), or mussels.

MAKES 4 SERVINGS

calories per serving	127	carbohydrate	25 g (78%)
cholesterol	0	sodium	65 mg
fat	.9 g (6%)	caloric density	30
protein	5 g (16%)		

CURRY SAUCE

2 cups Basic Chicken Stock, defatted (see index for recipe)
2 tablespoons whole wheat flour
2 tablespoons cornstarch
1 cup skim milk
¼ cup unsweetened apple juice concentrate
¼ teaspoon ground ginger
¼ teaspoon garlic powder
1 tablespoon mild curry powder or 1–1½ teaspoons hot curry powder

1. *In a saucepan, heat chicken stock to boiling.*
2. *In a separate bowl, combine flour and cornstarch. Add skim milk and apple juice concentrate and mix until smooth.*
3. *Add flour-milk mixture to heated chicken stock, stirring until thickened. Add seasonings and continue to stir. Remove from heat and serve warm or cool to room temperature.*

MAKES 12 SERVINGS

calories per serving	27	carbohydrate	5 g (77%)
cholesterol	0.3 mg	sodium	12 mg
fat	0.1 g (3%)	caloric density	47
protein	1 g (15%)		

SPAGHETTI SAUCE

2 15-ounce cans low-sodium tomato sauce or *1 28-ounce can*
1 15-ounce can low-sodium tomatoes, chopped, with juice
1 teaspoon dried oregano or *1 tablespoon fresh*
1 teaspoon dried basil or *1 tablespoon fresh*
2 tablespoons chopped fresh parsley
1–2 bay leaves
2 tablespoons dry red or white wine
1½ cups chopped mushrooms
1 cup finely chopped onions
½ cup chopped celery
3 cloves garlic, minced
*2 tablespoons Basic Chicken Stock, defatted (see index for
    recipe)*
Dash cayenne pepper

1. *Combine sauce, tomatoes, oregano, basil, parsley, bay leaves, and wine in a large saucepan and heat at medium temperature, covered.*

2. *In a separate nonstick skillet, sauté mushrooms, onions, celery, and garlic in chicken stock until tender (3–4 minutes, stirring frequently). Transfer to tomato combination and mix. Add cayenne pepper. Bring to a boil; reduce heat and simmer, covered, for 30 minutes. Remove bay leaves before serving.*

VARIATIONS

1. *Use 2 cups fresh tomatoes in place of canned.*
2. *Add ½ pound cooked ground lean flank or round steak for a spaghetti meat sauce.*

Makes 6 Servings

calories per serving	98	carbohydrate	20 g (82%)
cholesterol	0	sodium	17 mg
fat	.3 g (2%)	caloric density	30
protein	4 g (16%)		

CRANBERRY-ORANGE SAUCE

1½ cups fresh or frozen cranberries
½ cup unsweetened grape juice concentrate
3 tablespoons orange juice
1 teaspoon grated orange peel
½ teaspoon ground cinnamon
Orange wedges

1. *Heat cranberries, grape juice, orange juice, orange peel, and cinnamon in saucepan over medium heat to boiling. Cook until thickened (4–5 minutes), stirring frequently.*

2. *Remove from heat and add small orange wedges. Refrigerate for 30 minutes. Serve warm or refrigerate for 30 more minutes and serve cold over chicken, turkey, pancakes, or French toast.*

MAKES 6 SERVINGS

calories per serving	52	carbohydrate	12 g (92%)
cholesterol	0	sodium	6 mg
fat	0.1 g (2%)	caloric density	47
protein	0.2 g (2%)		

BASIC GLAZE

Use this glaze for making pies, fruit toppings, or fruit glazes.

⅓ cup unsweetened apple juice concentrate
2 tablespoons cornstarch
½ cup water

1. *Heat apple juice in a saucepan over medium heat.*
2. *Separately, combine cornstarch and water. Mix until smooth. Add to heated apple juice concentrate, stirring frequently. Continue to stir until glaze turns opaque and thickens. Reduce heat.*

VARIATIONS

1. *Add frozen or fresh fruit (approximately 3 cups).*
2. *Add to plain nonfat yogurt and fresh fruit to make a flavored parfait.*

MAKES 4 SERVINGS

calories per serving	54	carbohydrate	13 g (96%)
cholesterol	0	sodium	6 mg
fat	0.1 g (2%)	caloric density	64
protein	0.2 g (2%)		

17

LIGHT ENTREES: A LITTLE BIT GOES A LONG WAY

Traditionally, the entree has been considered the star feature on the dinner plate. Generally, it consisted of large amounts of animal-based foods such as steak, poultry, organ meat, or fish. On the grazing menu plan, however, the entree plays second fiddle to the tempting and tantalizing soups, salads, hot breads, and desserts. This revolutionary change is a result primarily of the concern over high fat, high cholesterol, and high calorie intakes in the standard American diet.

This chapter presents a selection of light entrees that include vegetables, grains, and small amounts of animal-based foods. Animal-protein foods are used occasionally as a condiment or flavor enhancer in our grazing recipes. Remember, these foods are higher in caloric density, containing more fat and calories per serving than their vegetable counterparts. The recommended portion size of cooked fish, poultry, or lean meat to 3 to 4 ounces a day. In addition, cholesterol is found only in animal products, whereas vegetables, grains, and legumes contain no cholesterol and are very low in fat content. Therefore, by increasing your intake of these healthful foods and by reducing your intake of animal products, you will be doing the very best you can to obtain a higher level of health and well-being.

Guidelines for selecting, trimming, and cooking with lean animal products are provided. Helpful hints for preparing foods without fat and cholesterol are also given. The entree recipes included in this section illustrate the method of stretching animal products without compromising elegance or flavor. Truly, you will see how "a little bit goes a long way."

GUIDELINES FOR PREPARING POULTRY, FISH, AND LEAN MEATS

Poultry

When using poultry, be sure to choose the white part of the meat and preferably the breast portion. Avoid the darker cuts of poultry. These have a higher fat and calorie content. Always skin poultry and remove the underlying fat deposits.

Fish

If you choose to include animal protein in your meal, the best choice is fish. On the average, the fat, calories, and cholesterol in fish are lower than in other animal products. Any choice of fish is acceptable on the L.A. Diet Program. However, some types of fish are leaner than others. For maximum weight loss, choose fish that are lower in both calories and fat. The following are good choices: cod, haddock, pollack, flounder, sole, turbot, halibut, red snapper, sea bass, sturgeon, brook trout, yellow pike, yellow snapper, and mollusks—scallops, oysters, snails, clams, and mussels.

The following fish are slightly higher in fat and calories and are acceptable for a weight maintenance program: bluefish, striped bass, catfish, carp, shark, swordfish, tuna, whiting, butterfish, lake trout, mullet, mackerel, lake whitefish, pompano, and salmon. There is some evidence that these fatty fish may have a beneficial effect on blood fat levels. Therefore, occasional use of these fish is perfectly acceptable on the maintenance version of the L.A. Diet Program.

There are a few special guidelines to follow when cooking fish:

1. When using fresh fish, cook for 8–10 minutes per inch of thickness (measured at its thickest point). This rule applies to any form of cooking such as poaching, steaming, broiling, or baking.
2. To counteract a "fishy" character, cook fish in an acid-containing liquid such as wine, vinegar, tomato-based liquids (salsa, sauce, or juice) or an orange juice, lemon, or lime sauce.
3. If using frozen fish, thaw in a refrigerator before cooking.
4. When purchasing fish, be sure the flesh is firm and has little or no fish smell. If the fish is whole, gills should be red and eyes bright and clear.

Red Meat

If you choose to eat red meat, there are two acceptable cuts that can be used on the L.A. Diet Program. Round steak and flank steak tend to be lower in fat than other cuts of beef. Remember, however, to eat red meat only on occasion because it contains a higher level of saturated fat than other animal protein foods (saturated fats increase the production of cholesterol by the liver). Limit portions to 3 to 4 ounces (cooked) per day.

GENERAL GUIDELINES

1. Trim all visible fat from poultry or meat. Remove before cooking to prevent fat absorption into other foods during the cooking process. Remove the skin from poultry before cooking.
2. To prevent drying out of the poultry, fish, or meat, prepare by methods such as poaching, steaming, stir-frying, or sautéing. Use an acceptable liquid as a base such as wine, defatted stock, vegetable juice, or water. Also, use high-water-containing vegetables such as onions, peppers, tomatoes, or carrots in the cooking process to provide additional moisture to the skillet. A process called "sealing" that retains moisture and flavor in your animal products is

achieved by quickly "stir-frying" in a small amount of liquid. This is popular in Oriental cooking and helps preserve the tenderness of your foods.

3. If baking or broiling poultry, fish, or meat, no liquid is necessary. However, to add moistness and flavor baste with an acceptable sauce or glaze.

We'll begin our entree section with a variety of fish-based recipes. These will be followed by several poultry dishes and other entrees using either little or no animal-protein foods.

FISH ENTREES

STEAMED SALMON WITH VEGETABLES

1 pound salmon steaks or any white fish, thawed
½ cup sliced onions
½ cup sliced mushrooms
2 cups broccoli flowerets
1 cup cauliflower flowerets
1 medium carrot, peeled and sliced
½ teaspoon dried thyme, crushed
½ teaspoon dried tarragon, crushed
2 teaspoons Worcestershire sauce
Lemon wedges (garnish)
Chopped fresh parsley (garnish)

1. Place fish in center of a large steam basket. Arrange onions, mushrooms, broccoli, cauliflower, and carrots around the sides of the fish.

2. Separately, combine thyme, tarragon, and Worcestershire sauce and brush mixture over fish.

3. Bring steamer to boil; reduce to medium temperature and cook, covered, for approximately 10 minutes. Serve with lemon wedges and fresh parsley for garnish.

VARIATION

Substitute poaching for steaming using ½ cup wine or water as the liquid base.

MAKES 6 SERVINGS

calories per serving	198	carbohydrate	10 g (20%)
cholesterol	26 mg	sodium	64 mg
fat	8 g (36%)	caloric density	129
protein	20 g (40%)		

BAKED HALIBUT AND PEPPERS

1 pound fresh or frozen (thawed) halibut steaks
¾ cup dry white wine
2 tablespoons fresh lemon juice
1 medium red pepper, seeded and sliced into rings
1 medium green pepper, seeded and sliced into rings
1 green chili, canned (rinsed), sliced into strips
¼ cup sliced onion
½ teaspoon dried dill or 1 teaspoon fresh
½ teaspoon no-sodium Italian herb blend
¼ cup chopped fresh parsley
Freshly ground pepper to taste
Lemon wedges (garnish)

1. Place halibut in a heatproof dish. In a separate bowl, mix all other ingredients together and arrange vegetables on top of fish.
2. Cover and bake in 350°F oven for 20–30 minutes. Serve each halibut steak with cooked vegetables and lemon wedges for garnish.

VARIATION

Marinate the fish and ingredients for 2 hours in the refrigerator. Broil fish and heat vegetable-marinade separately. Pour marinade over fish and serve.

MAKES 4 SERVINGS

calories per serving	133	carbohydrate	4 g (12%)
cholesterol	57 mg	sodium	96 mg
fat	2 g (13%)	caloric density	75
protein	25 g (75%)		

SEAFOOD CREOLE

3 cloves garlic
½ cup red burgundy or white wine
**1 pound fresh flat fish (cod, flounder, or sole) or any fish of
  your choice, cubed**
1 cup chopped onions
2 cups diced tomatoes
1 cup finely chopped green pepper
½ cup low-sodium tomato sauce
½ teaspoon hot pepper sauce (Tabasco)
1 cup sliced mushrooms

1. *In a large skillet, sauté garlic in wine at medium temperature. Add fish to skillet. Cook until fish turns opaque.*

2. *Add onions, tomatoes, pepper, and sauces. Bring liquid to boil. Reduce heat to low and add mushrooms. Stir once or twice. Continue to simmer, covered, an additional 10 minutes. Uncover and allow to simmer for 5 minutes more. Serve over long-grain rice or pasta.*

VARIATIONS

1. *Prepare without fish and serve as a vegetable side dish or sauce.*
2. *Substitute chicken for fish.*

MAKES 6 SERVINGS

calories per serving	94	carbohydrate	8 g (34%)
cholesterol	42 mg	sodium	66 mg
fat	1 g (10%)	caloric density	46
protein	13 g (55%)		

MAHI-MAHI ITALIAN STYLE

1 pound mahi-mahi or any flat fish
1 cup dry red wine
1½ cups Marinara Sauce (see index for recipe)
3 tablespoons diced green onions
Lemon wedges (garnish)

1. *Place fish in skillet. Add wine and cover fish with marinara sauce. Top with green onions.*
2. *Poach fish for 10 minutes until fish is tender in the center. Serve with lemon wedges as garnish.*

VARIATION

Bake fish for 20 minutes rather than poaching.

Makes 4 Servings

calories per serving	168	carbohydrate	17 g (40%)
cholesterol	70 mg	sodium	97 mg
fat	2 g (10%)	caloric density	46
protein	20 g (47%)		

CLAMS LINGUINI

6 cloves garlic, peeled and minced
½ cup red wine
2 bay leaves
1 teaspoon Italian seasoning
½ pound raw fresh clams or canned (rinse and drain)
1 15-ounce can unsalted whole tomatoes
12 ounces whole wheat linguini noodles

1. Combine garlic, wine, bay leaves, and Italian seasoning in a non-stick skillet. Sauté over medium heat for 3 minutes.
2. Rinse clams, discarding any that have opened. Shell clams and add to skillet; simmer, covered, for 5 minutes. Stir occasionally.
3. Chop tomatoes and add with juice to skillet. Cover and simmer 20 minutes.
4. Separately, cook noodles to al dente. Drain and rinse with cool water.
5. Serve clam sauce over linguini noodles.

VARIATION

Substitute scallops, oysters, or mussels (or a combination) for clams.

Makes 4 Servings

calories per serving	303	carbohydrate	55 g (66%)
cholesterol	30 mg	sodium	71 mg
fat	2 g (5%)	caloric density	90
protein	22 g (29%)		

POULTRY ENTREES

PINEAPPLE CHICKEN

2 medium onions, sliced thin
1 pound chicken breasts (4 halves), skinned and boned
½ medium red pepper, seeded and sliced thin
2 tablespoons Worcestershire sauce
⅔ cup unsweetened pineapple juice drained from can
2 tablespoons unsweetened apple juice concentrate
1 teaspoon grated fresh gingerroot or ½ teaspoon ground
*   ginger*
2 cloves garlic, crushed
1 16-ounce can unsweetened pineapple slices, drained

   1. In a heatproof casserole dish, place half of the onions on bottom of dish. Place chicken breasts over onions and top with remaining onions and red pepper slices.
   2. In separate bowl, mix Worcestershire sauce, pineapple juice, apple juice, ginger, and garlic. Pour sauce over chicken. Arrange pineapple slices over top. Cover dish and bake at 350°F for 40–45 minutes. Serve each breast of chicken over rice, pasta, or a bed of romaine lettuce and pour sauce evenly over top. Place two pineapple slices over each breast of chicken.

VARIATIONS

   1. To increase flavor, marinate chicken in glaze for 2 hours in the refrigerator before baking.
   2. Substitute 1 pound fish or acceptable meat for chicken.

MAKES 6 SERVINGS

calories per serving	151	carbohydrate	15 g (39%)
cholesterol	48 mg	sodium	95 mg
fat	2 g (11%)	caloric density	88
protein	19 g (50%)		

CHICKEN AND VEGETABLES

2 cloves garlic, crushed
1 cup dry white wine
1 pound chicken breasts, boned and skinned, cut into cubes
1 medium onion, chopped
1 cup sliced mushrooms
½ medium red pepper, seeded and diced, or ¼ cup pimientoes
1 whole canned (rinsed) green chili, diced
1 medium yellow squash, sliced
1 medium carrot, sliced
2 teaspoons grated lemon peel
1 teaspoon dried tarragon, crushed
1 teaspoon dried oregano, crushed
1 cup fresh or frozen (thawed) snow peas
Chopped fresh parsley (garnish; optional)

1. In a large skillet, sauté garlic in ½ cup wine over medium heat. Add chicken pieces, stirring frequently, until opaque. Add onions, mushrooms, red pepper, green chili, squash, and carrots. Continue to stir.

2. Add lemon peel and herbs to remainder of wine and mix. Add to skillet. Continue to cook, uncovered; reduce heat to simmer for 8–10 minutes, until most of the liquid is absorbed and vegetables are soft. Add snow peas during the last 2 minutes of cooking. Garnish with parsley (optional).

VARIATIONS

1. Use canned low-sodium white chicken (rinse) in place of fresh.
2. Add any variety of vegetables.

Makes 6 Servings

calories per serving	157	carbohydrate	12 g (30%)
cholesterol	49 mg	sodium	76 mg
fat	2 g (11%)	caloric density	66
protein	21 g (53%)		

HOT CURRIED CHICKEN SALAD

This salad can also be served as a sandwich spread or pita bread filling.

2 cloves fresh garlic, minced
½ pound boneless chicken breasts, cut into bite-size pieces
¼ cup red or white wine
1 cup chopped celery
1 cup sliced mushrooms
¼ cup diced green onions
1 8-ounce can water chestnuts, rinsed and sliced
1 cup Curry Sauce (see index for recipe)
¼ cup raisins
Dash paprika

1. In a large skillet or wok, sauté garlic and diced chicken in wine over medium heat, stirring frequently until chicken is opaque (do not overcook).

2. Add celery, mushrooms, green onions, and water chestnuts. Continue to stir. Cover.

3. Add curry sauce to skillet and stir until desired thickness is achieved. Add raisins and garnish with paprika. Serve hot with condiments such as diced apple, tomato, cucumber, and chopped bananas.

VARIATION

Prepare as a cold salad by adding ½ cup yogurt. Refrigerate 1 hour before serving.

MAKES 6 SERVINGS

calories per serving	135	carbohydrate	17 g (50%)
cholesterol	24 mg	sodium	65 mg
fat	1 g (7%)	caloric density	67
protein	13 g (38%)		

QUICK SPICY CHICKEN

1 pound chicken breasts, skinned and cut into strips
2 cups low-sodium salsa (to cover)

1. *Arrange chicken in a large skillet. Add salsa to chicken about ¼ inch deep. Add additional salsa to cover top of chicken. Bring to boil over medium-high heat. Simmer over low heat, cover, and cook for 10 minutes or until chicken in center is cooked. Serve with steamed corn tortillas or long-grain rice.*

VARIATION

Add ½ cup wine and additional vegetables of your choice.

MAKES 6 SERVINGS

calories per serving	116	carbohydrate	6 g (20%)
cholesterol	48 mg	sodium	18 mg
fat	2 g (15%)	caloric density	141
protein	19 g (65%)		

BEEF ENTREE

VEGETABLES AND BEEF ORIENTAL STYLE

2 tablespoons dry sherry
1 tablespoon Worcestershire sauce
1 tablespoon unsweetened apple juice concentrate, thawed
2 teaspoons cornstarch
2 teaspoons minced fresh gingerroot or 1 teaspoon ground
*   ginger*
3 cloves fresh garlic, minced, or 2 teaspoons garlic powder
3 large green onions, cut diagonally into large slices
½ pound flank or round steak, fat removed, cut into strips
4 ounces fresh or frozen (thawed) snow peas
1 medium yellow squash, sliced diagonally
1 medium red pepper, seeded and sliced thin
½ teaspoon hot red pepper flakes or Tabasco sauce

1. *In separate bowl, combine 1 tablespoon sherry, Worcestershire sauce, apple juice, cornstarch, and half the ginger, garlic, and green onions. Add the meat strips and mix to combine. Set aside.*

2. *In a large nonstick skillet (or use small amount of vegetable spray on a regular skillet), heat remaining garlic, ginger, and green onions in 1 tablespoon sherry, stirring frequently; reduce heat to medium. Add snow peas, squash, and red pepper, stirring until crisp-tender, 3–4 minutes. Move vegetables to outer sides of skillet, creating an empty area in the center.*

3. *Add hot pepper flakes to steak and marinating liquid; mix. Add steak to center of skillet, stirring until tender, approximately 3–4 minutes. Stir vegetables together with meat; reduce heat to simmer until ready to serve. Serve over long-grain brown rice or by itself.*

VARIATIONS

1. *Substitute chicken or fish for meat.*
2. *Add any variety of vegetables.*

MAKES 4 SERVINGS

calories per serving	163	carbohydrate	14 g (34%)
cholesterol	50 mg	sodium	76 mg
fat	3 g (16%)	caloric density	69
protein	18 g (44%)		

VEGETABLE ENTREES

QUICK AND EASY PIZZAS

¼ *cup Spaghetti Sauce*
4 *slices whole wheat bread*
¼ *cup nonfat or 1 percent low-fat cottage cheese*
¼ *cup sliced mushrooms*
¼ *cup shredded zucchini*
1 *medium onion, sliced*
½ *medium tomato, sliced*

1. *Preheat oven to 400°F. Spread 1-2 tablespoons sauce over each piece of bread. Add 1 tablespoon cheese and top with a combination of vegetables.*
2. *Bake for 10 minutes or until vegetables are tender.*

VARIATION

Use any of your favorite vegetables.

MAKES 4 SERVINGS

calories per serving	85	carbohydrate	15 g (71%)
cholesterol	0	sodium	168 mg
fat	1 g (10%)	caloric density	78
protein	4 g (19%)		

BEAN AND RICE SOFT TACOS

2 cups pinto beans, uncooked
1 tablespoon chili powder
1 cup long-grain brown rice, uncooked
1 cup chopped celery
1 cup diced green pepper
1 cup chopped yellow or white onion
1 teaspoon dried ground coriander
½ teaspoon grated fresh gingerroot or ¼ teaspoon ground ginger
2 cloves garlic, minced, or ¼ teaspoon garlic powder
8 6-inch corn tortillas
Low-sodium salsa or picante sauce
Shredded lettuce and diced tomatoes

1. Soak beans overnight in water. Add presoaked beans to crock pot with 6 cups fresh hot water and chili powder. Cook on high for 4 hours. Turn to low until beans are cooked. (Or cook beans in large pot over stove following directions on package.)

2. Separately, bring 3 cups water to a boil and add rice. Return to boil. Reduce temperature to simmer and cover for 45 minutes or until rice is done.

3. In a large skillet or wok, sauté celery, pepper, onions, coriander, ginger, and garlic until crisp-tender (approximately 3–4 minutes). Reduce heat.

4. In the oven, warm 8 corn tortillas for 10 minutes at 350°F.

5. Serve tortillas with a scoop of beans, vegetables, and rice. Top with salsa, lettuce, and tomatoes.

VARIATIONS

1. Add shredded cooked chicken.

2. For weight loss, add more vegetables than beans or rice. Freeze left-over beans for later use in other recipes.

Makes 8 Servings

calories per serving	180	carbohydrate	33 g (73%)
cholesterol	0	sodium	75 mg
fat	1 g (5%)	caloric density	117
protein	8 g (17%)		

FAVORITE ONE-POT MEDLEY

2 medium potatoes, washed and sliced
1 large onion, sliced
2 medium carrots, diced or cubed
2 cups fresh broccoli or 1 10-ounce package frozen broccoli
1 medium yellow squash
1 medium celery stalk, diced
2 cups fresh snow peas or 1 10-ounce package frozen snow peas

1. Place a steam basket in a large saucepan with ½ cup water. Add potatoes, onions, and carrots. Cook and steam at high temperature for 6 minutes or until potatoes are almost cooked (may need to add more water to saucepan).

2. Add remaining vegetables. Cover and continue to steam for an additional 3–4 minutes or until vegetables are tender but not overcooked. Flavor with salsa or a dash of Worcestershire sauce or low-sodium soy sauce.

VARIATION

Use any variety of seasonal vegetables.

Makes 4 Servings

calories per serving	122	carbohydrate	26 g (85%)
cholesterol	0	sodium	48 mg
fat	.3 g (2%)	caloric density	48
protein	4 g (13%)		

SUNRISE FRITTATA

¼ cup chopped onion
1 large carrot, peeled and sliced
1 cup broccoli flowerets
½ cup Basic Chicken Stock, defatted (see index for recipe), or
　　water
6 large egg whites
¼ cup skim milk
1 teaspoon Italian herb blend (optional)
1 tablespoon Worcestershire sauce (optional)
½ cup bean sprouts
½ medium tomato, diced
Low-sodium salsa

1. *In a large nonstick skillet, sauté onions, carrots, and broccoli in chicken stock over medium heat for approximately 6–8 minutes.*
2. *In a separate bowl, combine egg whites, skim milk, and seasonings. Mix but do not froth.*
3. *Spray a nonstick skillet with small amount of vegetable spray. Heat to medium temperature. Add egg white–milk combination, cover, and cook for 5 minutes.*
4. *Spread cooked vegetables over the egg base. Top with sprouts, tomatoes, and salsa.*

VARIATION

Make into an omelet by folding the cooked vegetables into the egg white–milk combination in step 2. Add to skillet. Turn to cook on both sides.

MAKES 2 SERVINGS

calories per serving	124	carbohydrate	15 g (48%)
cholesterol	0.5 mg	sodium	240 mg
fat	0.5 g (3%)	caloric density	34
protein	14 g (45%)		

ALBERTO'S ITALIAN EGGPLANT CASSEROLE

2 medium eggplants
2 cups broccoli stems and flowerets
1 tablespoon dried basil
2 teaspoons freshly ground black pepper
1½ cups Grazing Cream Cheese (see index for recipe)
1 medium onion, sliced
1 cup sliced mushrooms
1 medium green pepper, chopped coarse
6 cups Marinara Sauce (see index for recipe)
2 teaspoons paprika
2 tablespoons fresh parsley

1. *Slice eggplants crosswise into pieces ½ inch thick.*
2. *Sprinkle eggplant and broccoli with basil and black pepper and steam until slightly tender. Drain thoroughly.*
3. *In a nonstick casserole dish, spread a small amount of Marinara Sauce over the bottom. Alternate layers of eggplant with Grazing Cream Cheese followed by broccoli, onions, mushrooms, and green pepper.*
4. *Top casserole with Marinara Sauce. Sprinkle paprika and parsley over top.*
5. *Bake, covered, for 40 minutes at 350°F. Uncover and bake 10 minutes or until top is slightly browned.*

MAKES 12 SERVINGS

calories per serving	144	carbohydrate	19 g (53%)
cholesterol	5 g	sodium	65 mg
fat	2 g (12%)	caloric density	42
protein	10 g (27%)		

SUNNY MORNING POTATOES

4 medium potatoes, sliced
1 teaspoon garlic powder
1 teaspoon black pepper
1 medium onion, sliced
½ medium green pepper, diced
2 tablespoons white cider vinegar
2 teaspoons chopped fresh parsley

1. *Combine potatoes, garlic powder, and black pepper in nonstick skillet. Add 1 cup water and steam, covered, for 15 minutes.*
2. *Add onions, green pepper, vinegar, and parsley. Cover and simmer over medium-low heat for 10 minutes, turning occasionally.*
3. *Cook, uncovered, for 5 minutes to brown.*

VARIATIONS

1. *Add any variety of vegetables you choose.*
2. *Serve with low-sodium salsa or picante sauce.*

Makes 4 Servings

calories per serving	97	carbohydrate	21 g (87%)
cholesterol	0	sodium	8 mg
fat	0.1 g (.9%)	caloric density	65
protein	3 g (12%)		

18

BREADS AND GRAINS: FILLING UP ON HIGH NUTRITION

Hot baked bread, warm blueberry muffins, a steaming bowl of rice, and a hearty plate of pasta are just a few of the delicacies that await you on the L.A. Diet Program. Until recently, these foods were thought to be fattening and considered forbidden for those attempting to lose weight. Today, however, breads, whole grains, and other starches are considered a fundamental part of many weight-loss programs. When properly prepared, these foods provide valuable nutrients such as B vitamins, protein, vitamin E, trace minerals, and essential fatty acids. In addition, unrefined whole grains and starchy vegetables add fiber and bulk to your diet. They fill you up and satisfy your hunger without excess cholesterol, fat, sugar, and calories.

This chapter introduces many tasty high-carbohydrate recipes. These dishes can be enjoyed whether you're trying to lose or maintain your weight. Guidelines for adjusting portions for maximum weight loss are discussed. Methods for preparing cereals, breads, and grains are presented along with helpful cooking, storage, and serving tips.

CEREALS AND GRAINS

1. Experiment with a wide variety of cereals and grains, from the common ones such as rice, wheat, oats, barley, and corn to the more unusual—millet, bulgur, and buckwheat. Always choose grains in the whole form with the bran and germ intact. These unrefined foods are a more valuable source of fiber and nutrients than their refined counterparts. Look for whole grains in your local health food store or farmer's market.

2. Store grains in a cool dry place in airtight sealed containers. They should keep for approximately one year.

3. Recipes prepared with grains can be frozen in tightly sealed containers. Avoid keeping cooked grains in your refrigerator for too long before using. Otherwise, they can become tough and coarse.

4. As a time-saving measure, prepare grains in large quantities to use in meal preparation at a later time. They can be used as a breakfast cereal, lunch or dinner side dish, salad, soup, dessert, or entree.

5. For maximum weight loss, limit servings from the grains, breads, cereals, and other starches to four servings a day for women and six servings a day for men. Stretch grains in recipes by combining with lower-calorie foods such as vegetables. Grains can also be served as a garnish or finishing touch on soups or salads. This way you derive the flavor of the grain while reducing caloric intake to an optimal level for weight loss.

6. For maintenance of weight, simply eat cereals and grains to your appetite and caloric needs. For gaining weight, eat the starch-based foods to your heart's content, emphasizing the higher-calorie foods as opposed to the lower-calorie vegetables and salads.

7. Increase variety, flavor, and texture of your grains by trying some of the following suggestions:

• Cook grains in defatted stock, vegetable juice, or milk instead of water.

• Sauté onions, garlic, and other vegetables such as green

pepper or celery with raw grain kernels before cooking in liquid to increase flavor.

- Use herbs and spices during the cooking of grains or when sautéing the raw grain as mentioned above.
- Cook a combination of grains to intensify flavor and add variety. For example, cook brown rice with wild rice, barley, or buckwheat.
- Prepare grains for breakfast and flavor with small amounts of apple juice concentrate, raisins, or dates. Fresh fruits such as banana, apple, or blueberries and skim milk can also be added.
- To prevent grains from becoming mushy, avoid stirring before the cooking process is complete.
- If grains remain coarse after cooking, add a small amount of boiling water, cover, and continue to cook until sufficiently soft.

PASTA

1. When choosing pasta, look for varieties that are made with a whole grain flour such as wheat, corn, buckwheat, or brown rice. Some pasta is made with refined grain such as white flour or semolina flour, which lacks fiber and nutrients.
2. Avoid pasta and noodles that contain eggs. Read the label carefully to avoid additional fat and cholesterol.
3. Experiment with various shapes, colors, and types of pasta such as strands, twists, shells, lasagne, spaghetti, manicotti, and macaroni. Also, translucent noodles used in Oriental dishes make a nice light pasta. Avoid Chinese noodles that contain egg.
4. Follow package directions for cooking both pasta and noodles to achieve best results. Cooking times vary according to the pasta, but the end result should be *al dente* (not soft but firm to the bite). Noodles, on the other hand, should be cooked until soft.

5. To prevent overcooking, rinse and drain pasta under cool water. Avoid draining pasta too thoroughly to prevent stickiness.

BEANS

1. Beans differ in nutritional value, flavor, and texture. Experiment with the wide varieties available in your own grocery store. Store beans in a cool, dry place in airtight sealed containers. Cooked beans can be refrigerated for several days or frozen for later use.
2. Before cooking beans, rinse well and soak overnight. This helps reduce cooking time and may decrease the production of gas.
3. A useful method for preparing bean dishes is using a crock pot and allowing the beans to cook all day.
4. Add additional liquid such as water or defatted stock to the beans during the cooking process. Save the bean broth to provide flavor and thickness to other recipes. It's also a good source of nutrients.
5. The following suggestions can help make the most of bean cookery. Experiment and create some of your own favorites.

- Add vinegar, lemon juice, or wine to cooked beans to bring out a nice flavor. Lentils go well with vinegar, black beans with lemon juice. Begin with a tablespoon and add more to taste.
- Add herbs and spices to beans while cooking. Basil, bay leaves, cumin, celery seed, and dill are a few examples. Also, chopped vegetables such as celery, onions, carrots, and green pepper add flavor to beans.
- Combine several cups of low-calorie vegetables such as green beans, zucchini, carrots, and broccoli with the beans to reduce the caloric density. Starchy vegetables such as potatoes, corn, or yams increase caloric density and can be used freely for weight maintenance.

- To make a bean stew, add any combination of vegetables to the bean pot in the last half hour of cooking.
- Use left-over bean broth for preparing a rich gravy to serve over beans. The broth can also be used for making soups, stews, and casseroles.

BAKED GOODS (BREADS AND MUFFINS)

1. Use whole wheat flour in combination with yeast to provide a leavening action when preparing homemade bread. Baking powder can also be used in some breads, but avoid those containing salt. Use Featherweight low-sodium baking powder (available in most grocery or health food stores) whenever possible. Bread also requires kneading to strengthen the gluten.

2. Fresh yeast will keep for two or three days wrapped in plastic and stored in the refrigerator, though it should be used as soon as possible. In contrast, dried yeast will keep for six months in a sealed container. Fresh yeast should be dissolved in warm water before combining with other ingredients, whereas dry yeast should be sprinkled on the water. More heat and moisture are needed with dry than with fresh. Since yeast feeds on sugar, producing alcohol and carbon dioxide, 1–2 tablespoons of apple juice concentrate, date sugar, or barley malt can be used as the "food source."

3. Use whole wheat pastry flour (made from soft wheat) for recipes that require a lighter texture, such as pancakes, cakes, and pie crusts.

4. Blending whole wheat flour and a white flour helps produce a lighter product. White flour lacks nutrients but can be used in small amounts for this purpose. Rice flour or other non-gluten-containing flours can also be used.

5. When making quick breads or muffins, combine all dry ingredients first, mixing thoroughly.

6. Instead of using oil in muffins and baked goods, add fruit such as bananas, blueberries, apples, or applesauce as a source of moisture. In savory breads such as cornbread, use pimiento, whole corn kernels, or zucchini.

7. Unsweetened apple juice concentrate (thawed) is used as our sweetener. It is calorically less dense than other sweeteners, while providing a nice flavor.

8. Pure extracts such as vanilla, orange, maple, coconut, etc., provide flavor and essence. Avoid imitation extracts as they contain sweeteners, food colorings, and artificial additives and preservatives.

9. Use nonstick baking pans, muffin tins, and cookie sheets to prevent sticking. Also, spray a small amount of vegetable spray over pans for added protection. Avoid using paper muffin cups to prevent baked goods from sticking to the liners. The absence of oil in the recipes renders the cups useless.

10. In recipes calling for eggs, use 2 egg whites in exchange for each whole egg.

COOKING METHODS FOR BASIC STAPLES

1. Rinse grain in cold water and drain well.
2. Bring liquid (water, stock, vegetable juice, or other broth) to a boil.
3. Add grain slowly, stirring occasionally.
4. Bring water to a boil again.
5. Reduce heat to the lowest temperature. Cover. Cook until moisture is absorbed.

Beans and Peas

1. Rinse legumes in cold water. Soak overnight. Discard liquid the next day.
2. Cover beans with water, bring to a boil, reduce temperature to simmer. Cook beans, partially covered, until tender.

DR. JAY'S BLUEBERRY OAT BRAN MUFFINS

These are tasty enough to satisfy anyone's palate. Serve warmed with fresh fruit and herb tea for an enjoyable breakfast treat.

2 cups whole wheat flour
2 cups oat bran
2 tablespoons low-sodium baking powder
1¼ cups skim milk
4 egg whites
¼ cup unsweetened apple juice concentrate
12 ounces unsweetened frozen (unthawed) blueberries

1. Preheat oven to 350°F. Mix dry ingredients in a large bowl. In a separate bowl, combine milk, egg whites, and apple juice concentrate. Stir into dry ingredients. Avoid overmixing.

2. Fold in blueberries (unthawed).

3. Bake for 25 minutes at 350°F or until lightly browned.

VARIATION

Add diced apple, banana, or other fruit.

MAKES 18 MUFFINS

calories per muffin	104	carbohydrate	21 g (81%)
cholesterol	0	sodium	23 mg
fat	1 g (8%)	caloric density	166
protein	2 g (8%)		

EVERYDAY BRAN MUFFINS

¾ *cup whole wheat flour*
¾ *cup unbleached flour*
1½ *cups unprocessed bran*
1 *tablespoon low-sodium baking powder*
2 *teaspoons ground cinnamon*
1 *teaspoon ground nutmeg*
½ *cup raisins*
3 *egg whites*
½ *cup unsweetened apple juice concentrate*
½ *cup buttermilk (add 2 teaspoons lemon juice to ½ cup skim milk)*
½ *cup water*
1 *medium ripe banana, mashed*
1 *teaspoon vanilla extract*

1. *Preheat oven to 375°F. Combine dry ingredients and mix. In a separate bowl, mix liquid ingredients. Add to dry mixture, stirring approximately 20 strokes until moistened (avoid overmixing to prevent flat muffins).*

2. *Spray muffin tins with vegetable spray. Spoon batter into tins about one-half full. Bake for 15 minutes. Check muffins with wooden toothpick to be sure baking is complete. Remove and cool muffins on wire rack. Serve warm or store in plastic bags for later use.*

VARIATION

Add additional fruit (apple, blueberries, dried fruit) or grated carrot.

MAKES 24 MUFFINS

calories per muffin	64	carbohydrate	13 g (81%)
cholesterol	0 mg	sodium	11 mg
fat	0.3 g (4%)	caloric density	180
protein	2 g (12%)		

CORN BREAD

1½ cups yellow cornmeal
½ cup whole wheat flour
2 tablespoons low-sodium baking powder
1⅓ cups nonfat buttermilk (add 1½ tablespoons lemon juice to
  1⅓ cup skim milk)
3 egg whites
¼ cup unsweetened apple juice concentrate
½ cup canned, diced green chilies, rinsed

1. Preheat oven to 425°F. Combine dry ingredients in a bowl and mix well. In a separate bowl, beat buttermilk, egg whites, and apple juice together. Mix with dry ingredients. Fold chilies into batter; mix lightly until batter is smooth.

2. Apply a small amount of vegetable spray to a 10-inch pie plate and pour batter. Bake at 425°F for 25–30 minutes or until bread pulls away from sides of pan and top is slightly browned. Cool on wire rack. Serve slightly warm or wrap in plastic for later use.

VARIATIONS

1. Add additional vegetables such as ½ cup thawed corn, shredded zucchini, or grated carrot.

2. Use muffin pans for making corn muffins.

3. Add 1 cup blueberries to batter in place of chilies for a lovely breakfast bread.

MAKES 10 SERVINGS

calories per serving	111	carbohydrate	22 g (79%)
cholesterol	0.5 mg	sodium	5 mg
fat	.7 g (6%)	caloric density	170
protein	4 g (14%)		

OATMEAL PANCAKES

1½ cups rolled oats, uncooked
1 teaspoon low-sodium baking powder
1 teaspoon ground cinnamon
2 egg whites
1 cup skim milk
1 tablespoon unsweetened apple juice concentrate

1. *Blend oats in a food processor or blender until a flour consistency is formed (30 seconds). Add baking powder and cinnamon to processor and mix (10 seconds).*

2. *In a separate bowl, combine egg whites, skim milk, and apple juice. Add to the dry ingredients and blend until moist (or combine in bowl and mix by hand).*

3. *Apply a small amount of vegetable spray to a nonstick skillet and heat at medium temperature. Spoon about 3 tablespoons of batter on skillet for each pancake. Cook until bubbles form on surface and bottom is slightly browned. Turn pancake and cook other side until lightly browned. Avoid cooking at high temperature. Serve immediately with fruit topping, glaze, or sauce (see chapter 16).*

VARIATIONS

1. *To create "buttermilk" pancakes, add buttermilk in place of milk.*

2. *To make whole wheat pancakes, use 1 cup whole wheat flour in place of oats.*

3. *To make fruit-style pancakes, add ½ cup thawed blueberries, strawberries, mashed banana, or chopped apple or applesauce.*

MAKES 8 4-INCH PANCAKES

calories per 2-pancake serving	160	carbohydrate	26 g (65%)
cholesterol	1 mg	sodium	57 mg
fat	2 g (11%)	caloric density	143
protein	9 g (22%)		

FRENCH TOAST

4 egg whites
½ cup skim milk
1 teaspoon vanilla
1 teaspoon ground cinnamon
½ teaspoon grated orange rind (optional)
4 slices whole wheat bread, cut diagonally

1. *In a bowl, beat egg whites until frothy. Add milk, vanilla, cinnamon, and rind and mix with fork. Dip bread slices in mixture, turning on both sides until well coated.*

2. *Spray a nonstick skillet with a small amount of vegetable spray. Cook bread over medium heat, covered. Turn bread after underside is slightly brown and continue to cook, covered, until other side is browned. Serve warm with fresh fruit topping or fruit syrup (see Chapter 16).*

VARIATIONS

1. *Bake French toast in a 350°F oven for approximately 10 minutes on each side.*

2. *For a fancy-style French toast, add ⅓ cup plain nonfat yogurt and 2 tablespoons apple juice concentrate.*

MAKES 4 SERVINGS

calories per serving	85	carbohydrate	14 g (66%)
cholesterol	0.5 mg	sodium	183 mg
fat	1 g (10%)	caloric density	105
protein	5 g (23%)		

BASIC CREPE RECIPE

1 cup whole wheat flour, sifted, or whole wheat pastry flour
1 cup nonfat milk
¼–½ cup low-sodium carbonated water (e.g., Perrier or
  Canada Dry low-sodium club soda or seltzer water)
4 egg whites
1 teaspoon unsweetened apple juice concentrate

1. *Combine all ingredients in a food processor or blender. Mix until batter is smooth. Store batter in airtight sealed containers if not using right away.*

2. *To prepare crepes, spray a 6-inch skillet with a small amount of vegetable spray. Spray the skillet before making each crepe. Mix batter well. Pour ¼ cup batter into heated skillet, tilting to thin batter and cover bottom of pan. Cook over medium heat.*

3. *When bubbles form on surface and edges brown slightly, turn with spatula and briefly brown other side.*

4. *Remove from heat. Serve with filling of your choice—vegetables, fruit, nonfat cheese, etc. Roll to form a package. Top with sauce of your choice, if desired. To store crepes, place each prepared crepe between sheets of waxed paper or parchment paper and stack. Freeze in a sealed plastic bag or freezer paper for later use. To defrost crepe, place in microwave for 2 minutes or conventional oven for 5–7 minutes.*

Makes 8 Crepes

calories per crepe	70	carbohydrate	12 g (69%)
cholesterol	0.5 mg	sodium	41 mg
fat	0.3 g (4%)	caloric density	88
protein	5 g (23%)		

EARLY MORNING OATMEAL

⅓ cup old-fashioned rolled oats
¾ cup water
Skim milk to taste (optional)

1. *Combine oats and water in a small saucepan. Bring to a boil. Reduce heat to medium-low; cover and stir occasionally until creamy consistency is formed. Add skim milk in the last few minutes of cooking for a creamier consistency if desired.*

VARIATIONS

To the above recipe, add any of the following alone or in combination.
1. Vanilla Oatmeal: *Add ¼ teaspoon pure vanilla extract. Mix well.*
2. Almond Oatmeal: *Add 3–4 drops of pure almond extract. Mix well.*
3. Cinnamon Oatmeal: *Add ¼ teaspoon ground cinnamon. Mix well.*
4. Nutmeg Oatmeal: *Add ⅛ teaspoon ground nutmeg. Mix well.*
5. Fruit Oatmeal: *Add ½ banana, 1 chopped apple, or 2 tablespoons raisins or dates.*
6. Crunchy Oatmeal: *Sprinkle 2 tablespoons Grapenuts over cooked oatmeal.*

MAKES 1 SERVING

calories per serving	108	carbohydrate	19 g (70%)
cholesterol	0	sodium	1 mg
fat	2 g (16%)	caloric density	62
protein	4 g (14%)		

SPAGHETTI

1 pound whole wheat spaghetti
6 cups Spaghetti Sauce (see index for recipe)

In a saucepan, cook whole wheat spaghetti in water according to package directions. Serve spaghetti sauce over pasta.

VARIATIONS

1. Add clams, scallops, or other fish to sauce during the cooking to create a seafood spaghetti sauce.

2. To save calories, serve sauce over spaghetti squash or steamed vegetables instead of pasta.

MAKES 8 SERVINGS

calories per serving	230	carbohydrate	49 g (85%)
cholesterol	0	sodium	53 mg
fat	1 g (4%)	caloric density	67
protein	5 g (9%)		

BASIC BROWN RICE

1 cup long-grain brown rice, uncooked
2 cups water

Rinse rice under cold water and drain. In a saucepan, bring water to a boil. Add rice and bring to a boil again. Reduce to the lowest heat. Cover and cook for approximately 45 minutes or until moisture is absorbed. Avoid stirring to prevent rice from getting mushy. Fluff and serve.

VARIATIONS

1. Cook rice in 2 cups defatted chicken broth for added flavor.

2. Add diced onions, parsley, or other herb or spice during the cooking process.

3. Serve rice with a sauce such as an orange glaze or marinara sauce for a nice flavor addition.

• Time-saving tip: Double or triple the above recipe and make enough rice to last for a while. Store in airtight sealed containers and freeze. To reuse, thaw and warm in a microwave or heat rice with a small amount of water in a saucepan.

MAKES 2 CUPS OR 4 SERVINGS

calories per serving	65	carbohydrate	15 g (92%)
cholesterol	0	sodium	0
fat	0.1 g (2%)	caloric density	106
protein	1 g (6%)		

CRUNCHY RICE PILAF

2 cups Basic Chicken Stock, defatted (see index for recipe)
3–4 green onions, diced
1 cup long-grain brown rice, uncooked
1 cup chopped tomato
¼ cup nonfat milk powder
¼ cup frozen or fresh corn kernels
¼ cup chopped fresh basil or 2 teaspoons dried
¼ cup water chestnuts, drained
1 tablespoon Worcestershire sauce

1. Combine stock and onion in a large saucepan and bring to boil. Stir in rice. Reduce heat and cover. Simmer for 30 minutes.

2. Add tomato, milk powder, corn, basil, water chestnuts, and Worcestershire sauce. Simmer for about 10 minutes or until rice is tender.

VARIATION

Reduce rice to ½ cup and add ½ cup wild rice for a gourmet flair and nutty flavor.

MAKES 4 SERVINGS

calories per serving	132	carbohydrate	25 g (76%)
cholesterol	0.8 mg	sodium	63 mg
fat	0.4 g (3%)	caloric density	61
protein	6 g (18%)		

SPICY SPANISH RICE

1 cup long-grain brown rice, uncooked
1 clove garlic, minced
2 cups Basic Chicken Stock, dafatted (see index for recipe)
1 medium onion, sliced
1 15-ounce can low-sodium tomatoes, chopped, with juice
½ cup low-sodium salsa or picante sauce
¾ teaspoon chili powder
½ teaspoon dried basil
1 medium green pepper, seeded and chopped

1. *In a large skillet over medium heat, brown the rice and garlic in a small amount of stock (approximately 2–3 tablespoons). Add the remaining stock and bring to a boil. Reduce heat to low, cover, and cook for 15 minutes.*
2. *Add remaining ingredients except for green pepper and continue to cook for 20 minutes. Add green pepper and simmer for 10 minutes or until rice is well cooked.*

VARIATION

Add 3½ ounces diced white chicken breast or fish.

MAKES 8 ½-CUP SERVINGS

càlories per serving	104	carbohydrate	22.5 g (86%)
cholesterol	0 mg	sodium	37 mg
fat	0.5 g (4%)	caloric density	77
protein	2.5 g (9%)		

TASTY FRUIT AND RICE

2 cups cooked long-grain brown rice
¼–½ cup skim milk
1 tablespoon unsweetened apple juice concentrate
1 teaspoon pure vanilla extract (optional)
1 teaspoon ground cinnamon
Fruit of choice, such as 1 apple, cored and grated; 1 banana,
** diced; 2 tablespoons raisins; ½–1 cup blueberries**

Mix ingredients with cooked rice. Add fruit of your choice.

MAKES 4 SERVINGS

calories per serving	151	carbohydrate	33 g (87%)
cholesterol	0.2 mg	sodium	81 mg
fat	0.8 g (4%)	caloric density	99
protein	3 g (8%)		

19

DESSERTS: LIGHT, ELEGANT, AND SIMPLY DELICIOUS

The desire for desserts and sweets remains a never-ending passion for most people at any age. Whether satisfying an afternoon "sweet tooth" or completing an evening meal, desserts bring about enjoyable satisfaction. Why not have your cake and eat it, too? Indeed you can on the L.A. Diet Program. Desserts are part of the menu. However, the trick is in the method of preparation. On the American diet, desserts tend to be high in cholesterol, fat, sugar, and calories with limited nutritional value. Easy to overeat and difficult to resist, these desserts can be a danger not only to your waistline but to your health.

In this chapter, we explore light and elegant delicacies to enjoy on your new eating plan. Low in cholesterol, calories, fat, and sugar, these recipes provide more than sweet satisfaction. Many are valuable sources of nutrients such as calcium, vitamin C, potassium, and the B vitamins. Helpful hints and guidelines are included for preparing desserts. Enjoy these healthy treats and remember that desserts on the L.A. Diet Program can be enjoyed without one ounce of guilt!

NO-BAKE STRAWBERRY PIE

1 cup Grapenuts cereal or Nutri-Grain Nuggets cereal
2 medium bananas
⅓ cup unsweetened apple juice concentrate
2 tablespoons cornstarch
½ cup cold water
2 16-ounce packages unsweetened frozen strawberries (thawed)
* or 2 pints fresh*
1 teaspoon vanilla extract

1. *Layer a 10-inch pie pan with cereal. Slice bananas in thirds lengthwise and place over cereal.*

2. *In a saucepan over medium heat, bring the apple juice concentrate to a boil. Separately, combine cornstarch with ½ cup water. Mix until smooth. Add to boiling apple juice. Stir continuously until juice turns an opaque color and thickens. Consistency should appear as a glaze. Reduce heat to low.*

3. *Add the strawberries and vanilla to the saucepan; mix until glaze and fruit are well combined. Remove from heat and pour strawberry-glaze combination over cereal and banana. Let cool to room temperature. Refrigerate before serving.*

VARIATION

Use any fresh or frozen combinations of fruit.

MAKES 10 SERVINGS

calories per serving	104	carbohydrate	17 g (65%)
cholesterol	0	sodium	82 mg
fat	0.3 g (3%)	caloric density	81
protein	7 g (26%)		

ORANGE AND BANANA CAKE

1 cup raisins
¼ cup finely minced orange peel
⅔ cup 1 percent low-fat cottage cheese, rinsed and drained
¼ cup skim milk
4 egg whites
3 medium ripe bananas, mashed
1 teaspoon vanilla extract
¾ cup whole wheat flour, sifted
¾ cup unbleached flour
2 teaspoons low-sodium baking powder
1 teaspoon baking soda

1. Preheat oven to 350°F. Combine raisins and orange peel in a blender or food processor and puree. Add cottage cheese and skim milk; blend until smooth. Add egg whites one at a time and continue to blend. Add mashed bananas and vanilla.

2. In a separate bowl, sift flour; add baking powder and soda; mix. Fold flour combination into fruit and cottage cheese combination and blend lightly. Spray a bundt pan or deep baking dish with vegetable spray. Pour mixture into pan and bake at 350°F for 35–40 minutes. Cool on a wire rack. Serve warmed or at room temperature.

VARIATIONS

1. Use other fruits or fruit combinations of your choice in ¾ cup allotments.

2. To make muffins or tea cakes, add mixture to nonstick sprayed muffin tins.

3. Serve with a fruit glaze (see Chapter 16).

Makes 15 Servings

calories per serving	114	carbohydrate	22 g (77%)
cholesterol	0.4 mg	sodium	78 mg
fat	1 g (7%)	caloric density	184
protein	4 g (14%)		

CHEESECAKE WITH FRUIT TOPPING

½ cup Grapenuts cereal or Nutri-Grain Nuggets cereal
2–3 tablespoons unsweetened apple juice concentrate
2 cups nonfat or 1 percent low-fat cottage cheese, drained
½ cup nonfat plain yogurt
2 teaspoons lemon juice
1 teaspoon vanilla
2 egg whites
¼ cup frozen orange juice concentrate, thawed
2 medium ripe bananas, sliced

1. *Preheat oven to 350° F. Blend cereal in a blender or food processor until well refined. Transfer cereal to a bowl and add apple juice concentrate. Mix well to moisten cereal and pat firmly into a 10-inch pie pan. Prebake pie crust for 10 minutes at 350° F. Cool until ready to use.*

2. *Blend cheese, yogurt, lemon juice, vanilla, and egg whites in a food processor or blender until thoroughly mixed. Add orange juice and bananas. Blend until mixture is creamy (2–3 minutes).*

3. *Pour mixture over Grapenuts and bake at 350° F for 25–30 minutes. Cool and serve with the following topping.*

Makes 10 Servings

calories per serving (pie only)	151	carbohydrate	29.0 g (76%)
cholesterol	2 mg	sodium	105 mg
fat	.5 mg (3%)	caloric density	107
protein	8 g (21%)		

Topping

1 cup fresh or frozen (thawed) blueberries
1 cup crushed pineapple with juice
¼ cup unsweetened apple juice concentrate
1 tablespoon cornstarch
¼ cup cold water, cold or at room temperature

Combine all ingredients except cornstarch in a small saucepan over medium heat. Separately combine cornstarch with ¼ cup water; mix until smooth. Add to saucepan, stirring constantly until sauce thickens. Cool and pour over pie. To make a smooth sauce, puree ingredients in a food processor or blender before adding to saucepan.

VARIATION

For a variation in topping, add 1 cup of other fruit such as strawberries or other berries, peaches, or fruit of your choice.

MAKES 10 SERVINGS

calories per serving	36	carbohydrate	8 g (88%)
cholesterol	0	sodium	1 mg
fat	.08 g (2%)	caloric density	56
protein	.8 g (9%)		

BASIC SPICE CAKE

1 cup whole wheat self-rising flour, sifted
1 cup unbleached flour
1 teaspoon ground cinnamon
½ teaspoon ground allspice
½ teaspoon ground ginger
1 teaspoon low-sodium baking powder
1 teaspoon baking soda
1 cup skim milk
½ cup raisins
1 teaspoon vanilla
¼ cup unsweetened apple juice concentrate
2 large bananas, mashed
2 egg whites

1. Preheat oven to 350°F. In a large bowl, sift the dry ingredients together.

2. In a food processor or blender, blend the milk, raisins, vanilla, apple juice, and bananas. Fold liquid ingredients into dry ingredients.

3. Beat egg whites until stiff peaks form and fold into cake mixture; stir slightly but do not overmix batter. Spray a 10-inch bakers pan or tube pan with small amount of vegetable spray. Fold batter into pan.

4. Bake at 350°F for 30–40 minutes. Cool on wire rack.

VARIATIONS

Any fruit or vegetable can be added. Use the following measurements for each specific variation:

1. *Carrot Cake: 2 cups grated carrot*
2. *Carrot and Zucchini Cake: 1 cup grated carrot and 1 cup grated zucchini*
3. *Pineapple Cake: 1 cup crushed unsweetened pineapple*
4. *Date Cake: 2 cups pitted dates*
5. *Apple Cake: 4 large grated apples*
6. *Orange Cake: ½ cup orange juice and rind of 1 orange*
7. *Fruit Cake: 2 cups dried fruit*

calories per serving	147	carbohydrate	31 g (84%)
cholesterol	0.4 mg	sodium	60 mg
fat	0.7 g (4%)	caloric density	140
protein	4 g (11%)		

DELICIOUS FRUIT CREPES

2 tablespoons cornstarch
½ cup cold water
⅓ cup unsweetened apple juice concentrate
3 cups frozen or fresh fruit (strawberries, black cherries,
blueberries)
1 medium apple, shredded
16 crepes prepared from Basic Crepe Recipe (see index for
recipe)

1. Combine cornstarch with water and mix until smooth. Add apple juice and mix. In a saucepan over medium-high heat, bring cornstarch mixture to boil, stirring frequently. Fold in frozen or fresh fruit and shredded apple. Mix and remove from heat.

2. Warm crepes and place 2 tablespoons of fruit combination in center of each. Roll both sides of crepe toward center and turn over to hold in place (can also fold envelope-style). Serve warm with a dollop of plain nonfat yogurt or fruit glaze (see Chapter 16).

VARIATIONS

1. Serve fruit combination over pancakes.
2. To make a pie, scatter Grapenuts over a 10-inch pie plate. Dice 2 bananas over cereal. Pour fruit combination over bananas and bake in a preheated 350°F oven for 30 minutes.

calories per serving	197	carbohydrate	39 g (79%)
cholesterol	1 mg	sodium	87 mg
fat	.9 g (4%)	caloric density	72
protein	8 g (16%)		

YOGURT FREEZE

1 16-ounce package frozen unsweetened fruit (boysenberries,
strawberries, or blueberries)
3 tablespoons unsweetened apple juice concentrate
¼ cup nonfat milk powder
⅔ cup plain nonfat yogurt

1. *Place half of frozen fruit in food processor or blender and puree.
Add remainder of fruit and apple juice concentrate; continue to blend.
Add milk powder and yogurt and puree until smooth sorbet consistency
is formed. Pour mixture into a metal or glass container and freeze until
firm.*

2. *After fruit combination has frozen, put back into processor or
blender and blend until a creamy consistency has formed. Cover with
plastic wrap and store in freezer until ready to serve.*

VARIATIONS

*Substitute other fruit such as pineapple, banana, papaya, or mango
for a lovely frozen dessert.*

MAKES 6 SERVINGS

calories per serving	56	carbohydrate	11 g (78%)
cholesterol	1 mg	sodium	38 mg
fat	0.1 g (1%)	caloric density	51
protein	3 g (21%)		

CHILLED APPLESAUCED YOGURT

⅔ cup very cold applesauce
⅓ cup very cold plain nonfat yogurt
1 teaspoon ground cinnamon
2 tablespoons raisins

*Combine applesauce and yogurt. Add cinnamon and raisins and mix.
Serve chilled.*

VARIATION

Substitute ⅔ cup of any fruit (unsweetened pineapple, bananas, or blueberries) for the applesauce.

MAKES 2 SERVINGS

calories per serving	71	carbohydrate	15 g (84%)
cholesterol	0.6 mg	sodium	31 mg
fat	0.2 g (2%)	caloric density	47
protein	2 g (11%)		

FRUIT SORBET

2 cups frozen fruit, any combination (bananas are great)
1 teaspoon vanilla extract
1 teaspoon grated orange peel
2 tablespoons skim milk

In a food processor, blend 1 cup of frozen fruit. Slowly add the remainder of fruit, vanilla, and orange peel. Continue to blend until smooth. Add skim milk only if necessary to assist in smoothing the fruit combination.

VARIATIONS

1. Serve with Grapenuts or a dash of pure carob powder as a topping.
2. Add plain nonfat yogurt to fruit during the blending process.

MAKES 4 SERVINGS

calories per serving	83	carbohydrate	19 g (91%)
cholesterol	0.1 mg	sodium	5 mg
fat	0.4 g (4%)	caloric density	88
protein	1 g (5%)		

POACHED CINNAMON PEARS

1 cup red burgundy wine
1 cup water
2 teaspoons vanilla
½ cup unsweetened apple juice concentrate
½ teaspoon ground cinnamon
4 medium pears

1. *In a large skillet, combine wine, water, vanilla, apple juice concentrate, and cinnamon. Make sure ingredients are mixed well. Heat at medium temperature.*

2. *Peel pears, slice in half, and core, leaving stems intact. Add pears to poaching liquid and bring to boil. Reduce heat, cover, and simmer for 10 minutes, until pears are easily pierced. Remove pears and continue to simmer sauce, uncovered, until slightly thickened. Serve each pear with sauce.*

VARIATIONS

1. *Use apples or bananas in place of pears.*
2. *To prepare a flambé, add 2–3 tablespoons brandy to skillet, heat, and ignite.*

MAKES 8 SERVINGS

calories per serving	84	carbohydrate	20 g (95%)
cholesterol	0	sodium	6 mg
fat	.3 g (3%)	caloric density	55
protein	.4 g (2%)		

20
BEVERAGES

FRUIT SMOOTHIE

½ cup liquid (skim milk or unsweetened fruit juice)
1 medium frozen banana, sliced into chunks
½ cup unsweetened frozen berries of your choice

In a blender or food processor, blend liquid and banana chunks for a few seconds. Add frozen berries and continue to blend. Add more liquid if necessary.

VARIATION

To make a frozen sherbert, add less liquid.

MAKES 2 SERVINGS

calories per serving	87	carbohydrate	20 g (92%)
cholesterol	1 mg	sodium	32 mg
fat	.3 g (3%)	caloric density	56
protein	1 g (5%)		

HOT ORANGE CINNAMON TEA

2 cups boiling water
1 bag chamomile tea
1 bag Red Bush tea
2 cloves
1 tablespoon unsweetened apple juice concentrate
2 small pieces orange or lemon peel
2 small cinnamon sticks

1. Pour boiling water over tea bags, cloves, and juice. Let stand 2 minutes.
2. Strain and pour into two cups. Serve each with orange or lemon peel and cinnamon.

VARIATION

In step 1, add ⅓ teaspoon ground ginger.

MAKES 2 SERVINGS

calories per serving	26	carbohydrate	6 g (92%)
cholesterol	0	sodium	4 mg
fat	.02 g (.7%)	caloric density	63
protein	0.1 g (3%)		

ORANGE-APRICOT COOLER

3 cups unsweetened apricot juice
1 quart fresh or frozen unsweetened orange juice
1 quart low-sodium sparkling mineral water or club soda
Ice
Mint leaves for garnish

1. Combine fruit juices and chill.
2. Add mineral water and ice before serving. Garnish with mint leaves.

VARIATION

Add unsweetened fruit juices of your choice in the same proportion as above.

MAKES 12 SERVINGS

calories per serving	72	carbohydrate	18 g (95%)
cholesterol	0	sodium	5 mg
fat	.05 g (.6%)	caloric density	32
protein	.8 g (4%)		

REFRESHING FRUIT PUNCH

2 cups unsweetened pineapple juice
1 cup strawberries
2 cups unsweetened orange juice
1 cup low-sodium sparkling mineral water or club soda
Orange slices (for garnish)

In a blender or food processor, combine all ingredients except orange slices and puree. Pour into chilled glasses and garnish with orange slices.

VARIATIONS

1. *Add any unsweetened fruit juice and fruit of your choice.*
2. *Add ⅓ cup nonfat milk powder to provide a cream base.*

MAKES 6 ½-CUP SERVINGS

calories per serving	92	carbohydrate	22 g (95%)
cholesterol	0	sodium	2 mg
fat	.05 g (.5%)	caloric density	40
protein	1 g (4%)		

BASIC SPARKLING FRUIT DRINK

1 cup unsweetened fruit concentrate
1 quart low-sodium sparkling mineral water or club soda
Ice
Fruit slices for garnish

1. *Combine fruit concentrate and mineral water and mix. Chill.*
2. *Add ice before serving. Garnish with fruit slices.*

Makes 6 Servings

calories per serving	18	carbohydrate	4 g (84%)
cholesterol	0	sodium	4 mg
fat	.1 g (4%)	caloric density	9
protein	.3 g (6%)		

THE L.A. DIET EPICURE: A COOKING CLASS FOR MASTERING THE ART OF LIGHT STYLE ENTERTAINING

by Arlyn M. Hackett
Chef and Cooking School Instructor

We invited Arlyn Hackett, nationally known chef and cooking instructor, to write a chapter on entertaining and creating great tastes with light foods. What follows is an abbreviated version of one of his weekend classes in light style cooking. Instead of just demonstrating recipes, Mr. Hackett offers culinary principles for creating sensational flavors with light foods.

Mr. Hackett is a member of the faculty of the Culinary Arts Program of the New School in New York City. He also teaches at the Epicurean Cooking School in Los Angeles and the Pritikin Longevity Center in Santa Monica, where he was the chef for four years. His classes are offered in several other areas as part of an annual nationwide tour of cooking schools. He is the author of *The Slim Chef—A Cookbook for the Healthy Gourmet* and a winter holiday cookbook, *Can You Trust a Slim Santa Claus?*

—The Authors

Grazing on tidbits of food is not a new concept. For centuries the Chinese have had dim sum, little steamed or fried dumplings. The Spanish have their tradition of tapas bars, offering late afternoon snacks, typically accented with sausage. The English have tea accompanied by buttery pastries. Americans, with the advent of television, ritualized munching on cheese and crackers, chips and dip, and an occasional carrot stick. What is new about grazing with the L.A. Diet is the notion that all our eating should be light snacks eaten throughout the day and that those snacks should be high-fiber, high-carbohydrate foods.

Acceptance of grazing food depends on ease of preparation along with the ability to prepare appetizing dishes. People decide what to eat based on what they think will taste good. No one goes to the refrigerator and says, "I want 30 grams of protein, 40 milligrams of calcium, and 500 milligrams of Vitamin C." In the selection of food, taste is more important than nutrition.

To follow a weight loss diet successfully, you need to have food that tastes so good that you won't yearn for a forbidden delicacy to please your palate. This chapter shows you how to work with the appropriate grazing ingredients to create delicious dishes that need no apology for the absence of butter, oil, salt, or sugar—food so delicious that you, your family, and your friends won't even realize it's part of a weight-loss diet!

As a chef and instructor of light style cooking, I find it mandatory to offer my students more than just a collection of recipes. My goal is to offer a set of principles that will enable home cooks to bring great flavor to low-calorie dishes. Whether you want to plan a gala dinner party or just maintain your own epicurean standards, the tips and recipes in this chapter will help you make *delicious* synonymous with *nutritious*. What follows is a wealth of information that will help you enhance your repertoire founded in the preceding recipes to create fabulous dishes of your own—a cooking class devoted to light-style culinary concepts.

TASTING SOMETHING NEW WILL ADD 75 DAYS TO YOUR LIFE

This ancient Japanese proverb expresses the overall philosophy of this chapter: if you are going to change your life, then you have to be willing to try something new. This means trying unfamiliar foods, exploring new ways of seasoning, and using creativity and resourcefulness in the kitchen.

The following is a recipe I often use in my "Slim Chef" cooking classes. I draw attention to this recipe because it is one that students typically spurn upon hearing the ingredients but later, after actually tasting the dish, proclaim a culinary hit. You too may think blending a banana in vinegar a bit odd, but here is an invitation to approach cooking with a spirit of adventure.

NECTARINE COLESLAW

1 large nectarine, pitted
½ large banana, peeled
½ cup unsweetened and unsalted rice vinegar
¼ cup raisins
6 cups shredded cabbage

1. Combine the nectarine, banana, and vinegar in a blender and puree until completely smooth.
2. Toss the vinegar and fruit mixture with the raisins and cabbage. Mix until the cabbage is completely coated. Serve immediately or chill and toss again before serving.

MAKES 8 SERVINGS

calories per serving	41	carbohydrate	11 g (88%)
cholesterol	0	sodium	10 mg
fat	.2 g (4%)	caloric density	42
protein	1 g (8%)		

YOU CAN LEAD A MAN TO CARROTS, BUT YOU CAN'T MAKE HIM EAT

When one ponders what to fix for dinner, the first thought is not "I'll fix carrots." Rather, it is "I'll fix porkchops" or "chicken" or "hamburger" or "fish fillets" or "steak" or any number of possible meat dishes. Meat is the focal point of the American meal. And when it's not meat, it's cheese or eggs, which from a nutritional point of view may be even less satisfactory.

To get away from meat as the center of the culinary universe, I suggest that you think in terms of flavors. The focal point of the meal will be a particular flavor, such as curry, sweet and sour, spicy tomato, ginger and sesame, and so on. The flavor will be carried in a sauce. The sauce will accompany vegetables and a starch—pasta, potatoes, rice, or other grains. By starting with a sauce, you can create an endless variety of entrees that do not depend on meat for flavor.

When you're replying to "What's for dinner?" a "delicate curry" or "spicy marinara" is a more appealing response than "carrots." The following recipes for three sauces to be used over the same basic ingredients illustrate some of the diverse possibilities in light-style cooking. Beginning with a basic recipe of steamed vegetables and pasta, three sauces turn it into three distinctly different dishes.

Pasta with Three Sauces

BASIC RECIPE

1½ cups sliced carrots
1 cup sliced mushrooms
½ cup chopped green pepper
6 ounces dry soba buckwheat noodles (other egg-free, low-sodium noodles may be substituted)

1. Combine and steam the vegetables for 4 minutes.
2. Cook the noodles in boiling water for 3–5 minutes. Remove and drain.
3. Toss the steamed vegetables with one of the following sauces. Serve the sauce and vegetables over the pasta.

GINGER SAUCE

4 cloves garlic, minced fine
2 tablespoons finely minced fresh gingerroot
1 fresh jalapeño pepper, seeded and minced fine
2 shallots, minced fine
1 tablespoon low-sodium soy sauce
½ cup dry sherry
1 tablespoon finely minced fresh mint
1 tablespoon finely minced fresh cilantro
2 teaspoons sesame seeds, lightly roasted

1. Combine the garlic, ginger, pepper, shallots, soy sauce, and sherry. Simmer, covered, for 10 minutes.

2. Add the steamed vegetables from the basic recipe; heat through and toss with the mint and cilantro.

3. Pour the mixture over the noodles and sprinkle the sesame seeds over the top.

MAKES 6 SERVINGS

Nutrient data for each sauce, including the pasta and vegetables, are the same except for sodium:

calories per serving	139	
cholesterol	0	
fat	1 g (6%)	
protein	5 g (13%)	
carbohydrate	28 g (81%)	
sodium		
for the Chili-Orange combination	13 mg	

for the Tomato-Caper and
   Ginger sauces   110 mg
Caloric Density
  for Chili-Orange Sauce   87
  for Tomato-Caper Sauce 66
  for Ginger Sauce   92

CHILI-ORANGE SAUCE

¼ cup dry sherry
½ cup fresh orange juice
¼ cup unsalted vegetable juice
¼ teaspoon cayenne pepper
½ teaspoon ground cinnamon
¾ teaspoon ground cumin
1 teaspoon cornstarch
1 tablespoon lemon juice
1 tablespoon fresh tarragon or *1 teaspoon dried tarragon*

1. *Combine the sherry, orange juice, vegetable juice, pepper, cinnamon, and cumin. Simmer, covered, for 8 minutes.*
2. *Dissolve the cornstarch in the lemon juice. Add to the simmering sauce and stir until the sauce is lightly thickened.*
3. *Add the steamed vegetables to the sauce; pour the mixture over the noodles and sprinkle with tarragon.*

TOMATO-CAPER SAUCE

½ cup finely chopped onion
3 cloves garlic, minced fine
¼ cup dry red wine
1 14.5-ounce can low-sodium whole tomatoes in juice
1 tablespoon capers, rinsed and drained
6 leaves fresh basil, minced (1 tablespoon fresh tarragon or mint may be substituted)

1. *Combine the onion, garlic, and wine and simmer, covered, for 10 minutes.*
2. *Add the tomatoes and capers; simmer another 4 minutes.*
3. *Add the steamed vegetables from the basic recipe; heat through and add the minced basil. Pour over the noodles and serve.*

WHO SAYS YOU CAN'T MIX
APPLES AND ORANGES?

Another approach to deciding "what's for dinner" is to throw out the rules and redesign the structure of the meal. Where is it etched in stone that dinner has to be soup and salad, an entree with a starch and vegetable, followed by dessert? Why not make a meal out of four salads and dispense with the other items? Or how about a dinner with three kinds of soup? Would you consider a dinner of all appetizers? Grazing offers the cook wonderful opportunities for imaginative food presentation. Just don't be afraid to mix apples and oranges.

Most cooks view entertaining and a weight-loss program as incompatible. The diet is put aside when company comes to dinner. Providing a bountiful feast is synonymous with being a good host or hostess; a low-calorie menu fails to qualify as a "bountiful feast." If you are the kind of cook who wants to be slim but can't give up the idea of a bountiful feast, grazing fare was made for you! People who change to a high-fiber, high-carbohydrate diet are typically amazed at the quantity of food they can eat and still lose weight.

One of my favorite ways to entertain is to create a soup buffet. I offer three different soups with a salad and a simple fruit dessert. Soups have a hearty, comforting quality that satisfies both appetite and soul. By offering three soups, I give my guests variety with the option of being able to gracefully turn down a flavor that is not to their liking. The soup buffet creates an informal ambiance that promotes friendly conversation as much as eating.

The soups on a soup buffet should be varied but not incompatible. The following Black Bean Soup is a personal favorite. It combines a robust, hearty quality with a touch of elegance. Other soups that make good companions to the bean soup include tomato soup, corn soup, mixed vegetable soup, and the Spicy Borscht and Salmon Bisque included in this chapter.

BLACK BEAN SOUP

¾ cup dry black beans
5 cups water
1 large onion, chopped coarse
6 cloves garlic, minced
½ pound mushrooms, chopped
1 cup brandy
1 tablespoon low-sodium soy sauce

1. *Place the beans and water in a pot; cover and simmer over low to medium heat for 1½ hours or until the beans are tender.*

2. *Add the vegetables to the cooked beans along with the brandy and soy sauce. Continue cooking for 1 hour.*

3. *Remove the ingredients to a blender and puree until completely smooth. If necessary, add additional water.*

4. *Return the soup to the stove and heat through or reserve for later use.*

5. *Garnish the soup with your choice of bright-colored vegetables. Chopped tomatoes, red or yellow pepper slivers, celery leaves, cilantro sprigs, and minced parsley are a few of the possibilities.*

MAKES 8 SERVINGS

calories per serving	85	carbohydrate	16 g (71%)
cholesterol	0	sodium	50 mg
fat	.5 g (5%)	caloric density	32
protein	5 g (24%)		

YOU CAN'T FRY A CHICKEN IN WATER, AND YOU CAN'T STEAM ASPARAGUS IN OLIVE OIL

People on weight-loss diets seem to yearn for low-calorie dishes that taste like high-calorie dishes. The person who invents calorie-free chocolate is guaranteed to be a billionaire. Unfortunately, we still don't have calorie-free chocolate. As a chef my goal is to create low-calorie foods so delicious that no one need apologize for flavor. I believe I can create dishes without apology, yet I also accept that there are certain things I cannot do. I cannot make a chicken taste like fried chicken without frying it in oil. There are certain flavors that one will never attain with light style cooking.

Because oils and butter have become so integral to cooking, I find many cooks do not grasp the full range of what can be created with water-based cooking. Contemporary cooks depend on fat for both technique and flavor. Beyond steaming or boiling vegetables, most cooks are unfamiliar with such fat-free possibilities as braising in wine, stewing in broth, simmering in juice, or poaching in sherry. Settling for the ease of the microwave, cooks fail to develop other techniques that are light, healthy, and flavorful.

The cooking method is as important as the ingredients in creating flavor. To illustrate this in my cooking classes, I often ask my students to use a variety of different techniques to cook the same set of ingredients. The recipes below are excellent examples of how technique creates radically different flavors. Yam Salad Deluxe and Yam Stew Deluxe use identical ingredients. With steamed and raw vegetables the salad has a sharp, crisp flavor; the stew, with long and slow cooking, has a rich, sweet flavor.

YAM SALAD DELUXE AND YAM STEW DELUXE

1¼ pounds yams or sweet potatoes
2 fresh tomatoes
1 green pepper
½ large onion
⅓ cup champagne vinegar
3 tablespoons low-sodium tomato puree
1½ teaspoons curry powder
¾ teaspoon ground cinnamon

For Yam Salad Deluxe:

1. Peel the yams. Slice in ¼-inch slices; cut each slice in french-fry-size pieces. Steam the yam pieces for 5 minutes or until crisp-tender. Immediately rinse under cold water and set aside.
2. Cut the tomatoes in wedges.
3. Coarsely chop the green pepper and onion.
4. Blend together the vinegar, tomato puree, and spices.
5. In a large salad bowl, toss all the vegetables with the vinegar mixture. Serve at room temperature or chilled.

For Yam Stew Deluxe:

1. Peel the yams and cut in ½-inch chunks.
2. Finely chop the tomatoes.
3. Coarsely chop the green pepper and onion.
4. Stir together the vinegar, tomato puree, and spices. Add the vegetables and mix until the vegetables are thoroughly coated. Place the entire mixture in a baking dish and bake, covered, for 1 hour and 15 minutes at 300°F. The stew may be prepared in advance and reheated.

Makes 6 Servings

Nutrient data for both recipes are the same:			
calories per serving	154	protein	2.6 g (6%)
cholesterol	0	carbohydrate	37 g (92%)
fat	.4 g (2%)	sodium	15 mg
		caloric density	75

NOT ALL BROCCOLI IS CREATED EQUAL

The broccoli you buy today will likely not taste the same as the broccoli you bought last week or the week before. One may be stronger in flavor, sweeter, more pungent, or more cabbagelike. If, however, you put a little salt and butter on the broccoli, the differences in flavor rapidly disappear. Salt, sugar, and oils successfully mute, synthesize, and enhance flavors. When you omit the seasoning, you suddenly discover that not all broccoli is created equal.

When a cook seasons a dish, the goal is to make the dish taste better. The seasoning process can be broken down into three categories:

1. seasoning to enhance the flavor of the basic products
2. seasoning to synthesize the flavors of the basic products, thereby creating one new flavor, rendering the flavors of the major ingredients unrecognizable
3. seasoning to create contrasts in flavors

Seasoning to enhance flavor is the most common method used in American home cooking. A little salt and sugar are indeed effective in bringing out flavor. Without salt, sugar, and fats, most American cooks are at a loss for improving flavor. Creating a new flavor by synthesizing other flavors sounds appealing but without a specific recipe leaves most home cooks in a quandary. My experience as a cooking instructor in helping cooks break away from the salt-sugar-butter formula of seasoning is that seasoning by creating contrasts is the easiest and most immediately satisfying way of improving taste.

One of the most popular contrasts is that of sweet and sour. Other commonly used contrasts include sweet with bitter and peppery with aromatic. The following recipe uses all three of these contrasts. In creating a set of contrasts, the cook does not try to hide or disguise ingredients. Instead, one ingredient is used to highlight another while maintaining its own identity.

This may be understood more easily if you compare it to fashion and wardrobe. A yellow blouse next to a black and red skirt will appear vibrant and fluorescent; the same blouse next to a beige skirt will appear subdued. As for the black and red skirt, next to a gray blouse the skirt loses its flashiness and becomes formal and sophisticated.

In the following recipe for Spicy Asian Vegetable Salad, the jicama and papaya, both sweet, are a contrast to the sour vinegar. The two sweets also form a pleasant contrast to the slight bitterness in the vegetables. The mint, cool and aromatic, is a pleasant contrast to the spicy, hot pepper sauce. When I create a recipe, I try to create a variety of contrasts, much in the same way one builds a wardrobe.

A special note should be made about the use of herbs. Herbs offer a deep refreshing quality to most dishes, particularly when fresh herbs are used. This lively quality is frequently lost when dry herbs are used, and this is especially true when salt is not present. Dry herbs may have a slightly bitter quality that will linger on the tongue if not muted by the presence of salt. For example, the Tomato-Caper Sauce above will have a more pungent, slightly bitter quality if dry basil is used.

There are no rules for what to do or not to do, however. Learning by trial and error is in my mind the best way to learn the art and science of seasoning. In my cooking classes I often have my students create a variety of dishes using the same basic product as an exercise in the multitude of flavors that can be given to the same thing.

SPICY ASIAN VEGETABLE SALAD

½ pound jicama, peeled and cut into matchstick-size pieces
4 cups shredded Chinese cabbage
½ pound chayote, peeled and sliced thin
¼ cup canned water chestnuts, rinsed and sliced
¼ cup grated carrot
1 papaya, peeled and diced
½ cup low-sodium tomato paste
¼ cup rice vinegar
¼–½ teaspoon liquid hot pepper sauce (Tabasco)
2 tablespoons finely minced fresh mint

1. Combine the vegetables and papaya in a large mixing bowl.

2. Blend together the tomato paste, vinegar, and hot pepper sauce. Toss the mixture with the vegetable combination.

3. Just before serving, toss again with the fresh mint. Serve chilled or at room temperature.

MAKES 8 SERVINGS

calories per serving	59	carbohydrate	15 g (86%)
cholesterol	0	sodium	18 mg
fat	.3 g (4%)	caloric density	33
protein	2 g (10%)		

TOMATO JUICE WON'T
MAKE YOUR WALLS GREASY

A common complaint about low-calorie cooking is that it lacks richness—it tastes watered down. No matter how many herbs and spices are used to season the dish, it will still seem flat. Fats in cooking provide body and depth. Richness is usually achieved by adding such ingredients as butter, oil, cream, cheese, or other fatted products. A rich flavor can, however, be attained by using products that are fat-free but concentrated in carbohydrates and protein. Any concentration of calories will create a rich taste. The beauty of using concentrations of protein and carbohydrate is that the richness can be achieved with fewer calories. Purees of fruits and vegetables give depth and body while maintaining sound nutrition with plenty of fiber, vitamins, and minerals.

Other ways of adding depth include cooking vegetables in juices, broths, or wine (particularly woody wines such as vermouth, sauterne, and sherry). Nonfat milk powder and nonfat yogurt also provide depth and body. For flavor with almost no calories, extracts and essences are a bargain. A side benefit to these fat-free methods of providing richness is that they won't make your walls greasy!

In the Turnips and Apple in Onion Creme recipe, richness is achieved through a combination of a well-cooked onion, dry sherry, and nonfat milk. The Salmon Bisque has an amazing depth of flavor and richness, courtesy of the combination of broth, wine, tomato paste, yogurt, milk powder, and smoke flavoring.

TURNIPS AND APPLE IN ONION CREME

1 large onion
¼ teaspoon ground nutmeg
⅔ cup liquid nonfat milk
1 tablespoon dry sherry
2 turnips, peeled and sliced
2 apples, cored and sliced

1. *Place the onion in a covered baking dish and bake for 1 hour and 15 minutes at 300°F. Remove the onion. When cool enough to handle, remove the peel.*

2. *In a blender, puree the onion with the nutmeg, milk, and sherry.*

3. *Steam the turnips for 7 minutes; add the apples and steam for another 4 minutes.*

4. *Heat the onion mixture until hot, being careful not to overcook as the milk will curdle with extended cooking. Spread the onion creme across a platter; arrange the turnip and apple slices in the sauce.*

MAKES 8 SERVINGS

calories per serving	63	carbohydrate	15 g (84%)
cholesterol	.3 mg	sodium	40 mg
fat	.4 g (5%)	caloric density	35
protein	2 g (11%)		

SALMON BISQUE

1 pound salmon trimmings, including bones and skin
1 large carrot
1 large onion
4 cloves garlic
1 cup dry sherry
4 cups water
2⅔ cups plain nonfat yogurt
½ cup nonfat dry milk powder
2 teaspoons curry powder
⅛ teaspoon liquid hot pepper sauce (Tabasco)
1 teaspoon low-sodium soy sauce
¼ teaspoon natural smoke flavor

1. *Combine the salmon trimmings, carrot, onion, garlic, sherry, and water. Simmer, covered, for 3 hours. Pour the cooked mixture through a fine strainer or cheesecloth. Discard everything but the broth. Skim the fat off the broth.*

2. *Whisk together the yogurt, milk powder, and curry powder. When thoroughly blended, add the liquid pepper sauce, soy sauce, and smoke flavoring.*

3. *Stir together the broth and yogurt mixture. Heat through until hot, being careful not to overheat or leave on the burner too long as the yogurt will easily curdle and separate.*

MAKES 8 SERVINGS

calories per serving	66	carbohydrate	11 g (60%)
cholesterol	2 mg	sodium	112 mg
fat	.3 g (4%)	caloric density	33
protein	6 g (36%)		

IF A STRAIGHT LINE IS THE SHORTEST DISTANCE BETWEEN TWO POINTS, THEN SUGAR IS BETTER THAN HONEY FOR SWEETENING RHUBARB

In recent years sugar has gotten a lot of bad press. People have rushed to buy sugar-free products, unaware that the substitute sweeteners may not actually be any healthier. The major issue is not the kind of sweetener, but how much you use. Frequently sugar will sweeten a dish for a lot fewer calories than other sweeteners. This is not to imply an endorsement of sugar; rather, what is most important is to use sweeteners frugally and sensibly.

Sugar is an attractive sweetener because it is easy to use and because it is neutral, providing pure sweetness without imparting other flavors. Precisely because it is so neutral, it is often not the preferred sweetener to use. Consider the strawberries typically found in supermarkets. The berries are usually big, beautiful, and tasteless. Adding sugar only creates a dish of sweet "nothingness." On the other hand, marinating the strawberries in apple-berry juice concentrate or in diluted strawberry preserves will create richly flavored, sweet berries. Other fruits may likewise be enhanced by sweetening with juice or preserves. The juice concentrates and preserves should be only the kind that are fruit-sweetened.

Certain vegetables make an effective sweetener. Well-cooked carrots, onions, yams, or sweet potatoes when mixed with other vegetables provide a tinge of sweetness and successfully counteract any bitterness. Three centuries ago, before the widespread production of sugar beets and sugar cane, onions were commonly used to sweeten a variety of dishes.

Also in earlier times, dried fruits were commonly ground or mixed with water to create a syrup and used as a sweetening agent. Although calorically dense, dried fruit continues to be a nutrient-rich method of sweetening.

Nonfat milk, either liquid or powder, is another important nutrient-dense sweetener. By adding nonfat milk powder to yogurt, you can reduce or eliminate the acidic flavor of the yogurt. Adding skim milk to soups will produce a sweet, rich flavor.

A special way of sweetening is to create an illusion. Many products are so strongly flavored that when they are mixed with other ingredients you are unaware of the milder ingredients. In this way pineapple juice can be used as a sweetener for lime juice, lemon juice can be sweetened with orange juice, and apples will sweeten cranberries.

Not to be forgotten is the power of cinnamon and vanilla as sweeteners. Although generally considered for their own unique flavors, each used in small quantities will bring a touch of sweetness to a dish. For instance, a pinch of cinnamon will give a slight sweetness and will help curb bitterness in both a spaghetti sauce and a chili.

In the following recipes yams and onion are the sweeteners for the borscht, and apples, grapes, and cinnamon sweeten the cranberry relish. Elsewhere in this chapter, the Salmon Bisque is an example of milk as a sweetener, and the Marinated Strawberries illustrate the use of preserves as a sweetener.

CRANBERRY RELISH

1 cup whole fresh cranberries
1 cup whole seedless red grapes
1 large delicious apple, cored
1 teaspoon ground cinnamon
1 tablespoon grated orange peel

1. Combine all the ingredients in a food processor or food grinder and process until coarsely chopped or ground.
2. Chill before serving.

Makes 8 Servings

calories per serving	24	carbohydrate	6 g (91%)
cholesterol	0	sodium	1 mg
fat	.2 g (7%)	caloric density	58
protein	.2 g (2%)		

SPICY BORSCHT

3 beets, peeled and cut julienne-style
1 cup grated yam or sweet potato
½ cup coarsely chopped red onion
2 tablespoons finely minced fresh gingerroot
5 cups water
3 cups shredded red cabbage
⅓ cup vinegar
½ cup unsalted tomato paste
¼ teaspoon liquid hot pepper sauce (Tabasco)

1. Combine the beets, yam, onion, ginger, and water and simmer, covered, for 45 minutes

2. Add the cabbage and simmer for another 15 minutes.

3. Add the remaining ingredients, stirring to blend the mixture thoroughly. Cook for another 5 minutes and serve.

MAKES 8 SERVINGS

calories per serving	52	carbohydrate	13 g (85%)
cholesterol	0	sodium	28 mg
fat	.3 g (4%)	caloric density	43
protein	2 g (11%)		

ROME WASN'T BUILT IN A DAY, BUT THEN AGAIN, DO YOU WANT TO SPEND ALL DAY IN THE KITCHEN?

Most contemporary cooks want recipes that are quick and easy. The age of the microwave has produced the mentality that, if you can't do it in five minutes, order out. Preparing fresh products requires time. I personally believe the difference in taste and nutrition is worth the extra hassle. I also want to be realistic, however. Living a full life means more than living in the kitchen. The following recipes were created specifically for low-calorie, no-apology entertaining. The food, light and refreshing, is quickly and easily prepared. Cooking and preparation time for the entire meal should not exceed 40 minutes.

SUMMER SALAD

3 fresh apricots
1 head lettuce
3 green onions
½ cup plain nonfat yogurt
4 teaspoons low-sodium Dijon-style mustard
2 tablespoons apricot or peach preserves (fruit-sweetened only)
2 tablespoons champagne vinegar
½ cup canned water chestnuts, sliced

1. Cut the apricots in half and remove the pits; slice each half in 4 parts.
2. Carefully wash the lettuce and thoroughly dry with a towel or salad spinner. Tear the lettuce in bite-size pieces.
3. Chop the green onions, discarding most of the green stalks.
4. Combine the yogurt, mustard, preserves, and vinegar. Whisk until smooth.
5. Toss the lettuce with the yogurt mixture until all the leaves are thoroughly coated. Place the dressed lettuce on individual chilled salad plates.
6. Attractively arrange the apricots and water chestnuts over the lettuce. Sprinkle each plate with the chopped onion.

MAKES 6 SERVINGS

calories per serving	52	carbohydrate	11 g (80%)
cholesterol	3 mg	sodium	18 mg
fat	.4 g (5%)	caloric density	56
protein	2 g (15%)		

ORANGE ROUGHY IN LIME AND GINGER
SAUCE

3 cups boiling water
1½ cups brown rice
1½ pounds orange roughy (or sea bass) fillets
¼ cup fresh lime juice
¼ cup unsweetened pineapple juice
2 teaspoons freshly grated gingerroot
6 small sprigs of fresh cilantro (coriander)
2 teaspoons low-sodium soy sauce

1. In a small saucepan, pour the boiling water over the rice. Cover and simmer over low heat for 40 mintues.

2. Cut the fish fillets into 6 portions. Combine the juices and pour over the fish in a shallow pan. Add the grated ginger and marinate for 30 minutes.

3. Simmer the fish over medium heat for 8 minutes. Keep the pan covered while cooking.

4. Remove the fish to a heated platter. Pour the juices over the fish and garnish with sprigs of cilantro. Stir the soy sauce into the rice just before serving and serve the fish with the rice.

MAKES 6 SERVINGS

calories per serving	205	carbohydrate	27 g (54%)
cholesterol	29 mg	sodium	57 mg
fat	3 g (12%)	caloric density	108
protein	17 g (34%)		

MARINATED STRAWBERRIES

2 tablespoons strawberry preserves (fruit-sweetened only)
2 tablespoons water
2 cups sliced fresh strawberries

1. Combine the preserves and water in a small saucepan. Heat the mixture slightly and stir until the preserves are thoroughly blended.

2. Toss the sliced berries with the liquid and chill. Stir occasionally to marinate the berries completely.

calories per serving	47	carbohydrate	12 g (90%)
cholesterol	0	sodium	6 mg
fat	.3 g (5%)	caloric density	46
protein	.7 g (5%)		

Other dishes can be added to this party menu for those with higher-calorie needs. Consider serving a whole grain bread with pure fruit preserves, a steamed vegetable topped with a spoon of unsalted mustard, or yogurt on the side with the strawberries.

CHOCOLATE IS CHOCOLATE, AND CAROB IS CAROB

I am afraid that creators of diet recipes are often guilty of creating phony food—dishes that are supposed to taste like a famous high-calorie dish yet without the calories. I have yet to taste a "mock mayonnaise" that tastes like real mayonnaise. Carob is tasty, but it is not chocolate. That does not mean that carob is less tasty than chocolate; it is simply different.

High-fat dishes that have been changed to conform to light style standards face the prospect of being viewed as inferior. In replacing high-fat ingredients, it is important not to sacrifice flavor. Of course part of deciding what tastes good is predetermined by our expectations for a dish. If you have had traditional Celery Root Remoulade, made with mayonnaise, then you may be disappointed by the following recipe. On the other hand, if you have never experienced the traditional version, this new recipe with yogurt may not only please but be the preferred flavor.

To counteract the power of expectations, I suggest that you change the appearance and name of the adaptation. For instance, in the following version of Celery Root Remoulade, artichoke hearts have been added to give it a new look as well as a new twist in flavor. By changing the name to Celery Root Celeste, you don't remind diners of a previous dining experience that they will uphold as a comparison. The dish stands on its own merits and does not compete with past visions of mayonnaise.

CELERY ROOT CELESTE

1 celery root
1 cup water
1 10-ounce package frozen artichoke hearts
2 cloves garlic, minced fine
½ cup extra-dry vermouth
⅔ cup plain nonfat yogurt
3 tablespoons dry nonfat milk powder
2 tablespoons low-sodium Dijon-style mustard
2 drops pure lemon extract
2 drops (or more) liquid hot pepper sauce (Tabasco)
4 green onions

1. *Peel the celery root; slice in julienne strips. Place on a steamer rack above the water and steam for 8 minutes or until tender.*

2. *Combine the artichoke hearts, garlic, and vermouth and simmer for 8 minutes.*

3. *Whisk together the yogurt, milk powder, and mustard until completely smooth. Add the liquid from the cooked artichoke hearts, the lemon extract, and the hot sauce to the yogurt mixture. Stir until blended.*

4. *Toss the yogurt mixture with artichokes, garlic, and celery root. Top with the chopped green onion.*

MAKES 8 SERVINGS

calories per serving	53	carbohydrate	10 g (70%)
cholesterol	1 mg	sodium	89 mg
fat	.4 g (6%)	caloric density	46
protein	3 g (6%)		

I NEVER PROMISED YOU A ROSE GARDEN BECAUSE I WANTED YOU TO HAVE AN HERB GARDEN INSTEAD

People constantly ask me if I feel my creativity is stifled by avoiding the use of salt, butter, oils, cream, and cheese. My response is simply "No." We do not view the sculptor who works only in bronze as less creative or talented than the artist who works with metal, plastic, and wood. I view a restriction on ingredients as a creative opportunity that may result in flavors that would never have been discovered without a limitation of choices. Limited ingredients is no excuse for boring food.

I find that when a cook enjoys cooking, the diner usually has an equally enjoyable experience. If you are just beginning to change your style of cooking, I suggest that you relax, accept that every dish doesn't have to be perfect, and have a great time experimenting. Besides being pleased with the results of a change in lifestyle, I hope the process of getting there will also be pleasurable. Experimenting with fresh herbs from your own window herb garden, or trying different wines for poaching fish, or exploring a variety of preserves and juices as sweeteners will likely result in the creation of your own culinary masterpieces!

INDEX

291

NOTES

NOTES

NOTES

NOTES